Clinical Care of the Diabetic Foot

David G. Armstrong, DPM, PhD, MSc, and
Lawrence A. Lavery, DPM, MPH, Editors

D1319608

American Diabetes Association.
Cure • Care • Commitment®

Director, Book Publishing, John Fedor; *Associate Director, Professional Books,* Christine B. Charlip; *Editor,* Rebecca Lanning; *Copyeditor,* Mary Beth Keegan; *Associate Director, Book Production,* Peggy M. Rote; *Composition,* Circle Graphics, Inc.; *Cover Design,* Koncept, Inc.; *Printer,* Transcontinental Printing.

Printed in Canada
1 3 5 7 9 10 8 6 4 2

The suggestions and information contained in this publication are generally consistent with the *Clinical Practice Recommendations* and other policies of the American Diabetes Association, but they do not represent the policy or position of the Association or any of its boards or committees. Reasonable steps have been taken to ensure the accuracy of the information presented. However, the American Diabetes Association cannot ensure the safety or efficacy of any product or service described in this publication. Individuals are advised to consult a physician or other appropriate health care professional before undertaking any diet or exercise program or taking any medication referred to in this publication. Professionals must use and apply their own professional judgment, experience, and training and should not rely solely on the information contained in this publication before prescribing any diet, exercise, or medication. The American Diabetes Association—its officers, directors, employees, volunteers, and members—assumes no responsibility or liability for personal or other injury, loss, or damage that may result from the suggestions or information in this publication.

Ⓧ The paper in this publication meets the requirements of the ANSI Standard Z39.48-1992 (permanence of paper).

ADA titles may be purchased for business or promotional use or for special sales. To purchase this book in large quantities, or for custom editions of this book with your logo, contact Lee Romano Sequeira, Special Sales & Promotions, at the address below, or at LRomano@ diabetes.org or call 703-299-2046.

American Diabetes Association
1701 North Beauregard Street
Alexandria, Virginia 22311

Library of Congress Cataloging-in-Publication Data

Clinical care of the diabetic foot / [edited by] David G. Armstrong and Lawrence A. Lavery.
    p. ; cm.
  Includes bibliographical references and index.
  ISBN 1-58040-223-2
  1. Foot—Diseases. 2. Diabetes—Complications. 3. Foot—Surgery.
  [DNLM: 1. Diabetic Foot. WK 835 C6403 2005] I. Armstrong, David G., 1969– II. Lavery, Lawrence A., 1960– III. American Diabetes Association.

  RC951.C49 2005
  617.5'85—dc22
                        2004029087

To my beautiful wife, Tania, and our glorious children, Alexandria, Natalie, and Nina. I hope this work in some small way honors you for all that you have done to honor me.

—DGA

To my beautiful wife, Karen. Without your patience and support, little of my work would see the light of day. Thank you for taking care of all of us guys.

—LAL

Contents

Preface

"The era of coma has given way to the era of complications"

—Elliot P. Joslin

PROFESSOR JOSLIN'S QUOTE, from the first half of the last century, is as fitting today as it was some seventy years ago. Our patients with diabetes no longer die from acute conditions stemming from hyperglycemia. Rather, it is the chronic complications of the disease that predominate. Chief among these complications is pathology of the diabetic foot, which is the most common reason for hospital admission among people with diabetes. Only a generation ago, most clinicians considered it a fait accompli that people with diabetes who developed lower-extremity complications would face amputation, reamputation, and premature death. Over the past generation, care of the diabetic foot has matured from its previous state of nihilism into a bona fide area of subspecialty and hope. It is now widely accepted that many lower-extremity complications of diabetes are preventable.

Care of the diabetic foot spans the spectrum from surgery to endocrinology, podiatry to infectious disease, psychology to dermatology. While many clinicians appreciate that this area deserves attention, most are so focused on and inundated with more proximal issues that the myriad potential distal complications seem both daunting and beyond control. It is to these clinicians that this book is dedicated.

We are honored and humbled to have worked with such a stellar cast of clinician-scientists in the production of this book. It assembles under one cover many of the people collectively responsible for transforming and advancing diabetic foot and wound care from its beginnings into its current state. Together, these contributors discuss nearly all aspects of diabetic foot and wound care in a practical yet evidence-based manner.

To you, the reader, we extend an enthusiastic invitation to avail yourself of the collective wisdom of these contributors. We hope that this work will stimulate you to investigate further what we believe is a hugely fascinating and fruitful area of medicine. Enjoy.

David G. Armstrong, DPM, PhD, MSc
North Chicago, Illinois

Lawrence A. Lavery, DPM, MPH
Temple, Texas

The Role of Systemic Disease in Diabetic Foot Complications

Peter Sheehan, MD

Foot ulceration is a disturbing complication of diabetes that often results in a diminished quality of life. By a "rule of 15," 15% of people with diabetes develop ulcers, 15% of ulcers develop osteomyelitis, and 15% of ulcers result in amputation. Foot ulcers are costly, with a 2-year expense of nearly $30,000 per patient, and they account for about 20% of hospital inpatient days for people with diabetes. This figure is even more striking when one considers that 60% of all diabetes costs are for inpatient care. Thus, the economic impact is staggering.

When the outcome is amputation, treatment costs soar to nearly $60,000 per patient over the 2-year period. For the patient, the profound emotional loss of amputation resembles bereavement. Unfortunately, amputation is not the end of the story. Approximately half of these patients will have a contralateral amputation within 3 years—and half will die within 5 years. Admittedly, many of these people are moribund and at high cardiovascular risk, but the psychosocial effects of amputation may contribute to their demise.

Using a component model, Pecoraro, Reiber, and Burgess delineated the "causal pathway" to amputation with a landmark analysis of individual clinical factors in patients with diabetes. No factor alone was sufficient to result in amputation, but several in concert could. Nearly three-quarters of amputations had the following component pathway:

- peripheral neuropathy—an essential aspect
- trauma—usually from just daily ambulation
- ulceration—typically of the plantar skin
- faulty healing

In time, infection or ischemia may worsen, and patients succumb to amputation. Thus, the road to amputation is usually through a foot ulcer.

What constitutes faulty healing? Does it characterize all chronic wounds? And is it different in patients with diabetes and foot ulcerations? This introduction attempts to answer these questions as it reviews the pathophysiology of the chronic wound and of impaired cutaneous healing and discusses the local and systemic factors that uniquely contribute to the faulty healing of the diabetic foot ulcer.

The Chronic Wound

Pathophysiology of Acute Wounds

The pathophysiology of acute wound healing has been categorized as a hierarchical progression through four distinct phases. The first phase is *coagulation,* which occurs immediately at the time of tissue injury. The key cell activated in this phase is the platelet, which aggregates at the area of injury, binds thrombin, and forms a plug. In addition, vasoconstriction occurs and cytokines and growth factors—including platelet-derived growth factors and fibroblast growth factors—are released. These initiate healing and act as chemoattractants for circulating polymorphonuclear cells and macrophages.

With vasodilatation, these cells enter the wound and initiate the *inflammation* phase (Fig. 1). Here the inflammatory cells phagocytose bacteria, and macrophages produce more cytokines and growth factors, like interleukin-6 (IL-6), fibroblast growth factor (FGF), and

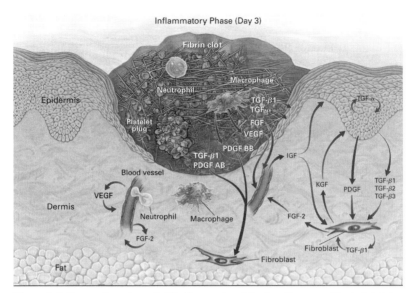

Figure 1 Inflammation phase. Infiltrating neutrophils clear the wound bed of debris and bacteria. The fibrin clot serves as a "provisional matrix" for macrophages which transform into an inflammatory phenotype, producing various growth factors and cytokines. These cytokines stimulate fibroblasts from around the wound, inducing autocrine and paracrine activity and promoting infiltration into the provisional matrix. *From* Singer and Clark, reprinted with permission. © 1999 Massachusetts Medical Society. All rights reserved.

transforming growth factor–β (TGF-β). Through paracrine and autocrine mechanisms, these growth factors serve as a call to action for fibroblasts, which infiltrate the provisional matrix and begin to produce the matrix components fibronectin and collagen. The inflammatory cells produce matrix metalloproteases (MMPs), enzymes that digest collagens and elastins, and components of the fibrin clot, or provisional matrix.

The MMPs also clear the way for endothelial cells and new vessel formation, or angiogenesis. In a sense they are "drilling for oxygen" for the healing wound. When this process finally occurs, the *proliferation* phase begins (Fig. 2). Fibroblasts and endothelial cells are recruited locally and from circulating precursors from the bone marrow, presumably drawn in by several of the angiogenic growth factors present in the wound. The newly formed matrix, with its rich arcade of new vessels, appears to the naked eye to be fine red granules termed "granulation."

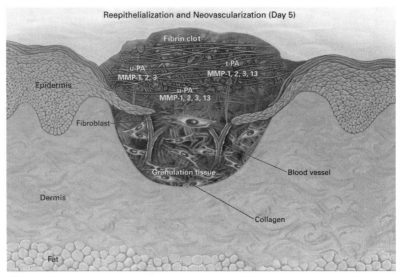

Figure 2 Proliferation phase. Fibroblasts infiltrate the provisional matrix and begin the creation of a lattice of fibronectin, collagen, and other components. In addition, they produce plasminogen activator (tPA) and matrix metalloproteases (MMPs), which allow the movement of endothelial cells into the wound. Hypoxia, lactic acid, and other factors support the angiogenesis and creation of granulation tissue, which is ultimately covered by migrating keratinocytes from the neighboring epidermis. *From* Singer and Clark, reprinted with permission. © 1999 Massachusetts Medical Society. All rights reserved.

This granulation tissue supplies a supporting lattice to allow the migration of keratinocytes across the surface of the wound to create a new epidermis. After re-epithelialization, endothelial cells undergo apoptosis, and the granulation tissue is replaced by collagen and dermal elements.

Simultaneously, scar formation and collagen shortening occur, and fibroblasts are transformed into myofibroblasts, causing the wound to contract like a purse string. When the wound is closed, completely covered with epithelium, and not draining, it is considered healed (a process that usually takes 10–14 days in an acute wound) and the *remodeling* phase begins. In this phase, which may continue for 6–12 months, the collagen fibrils in the scar tissue are remodeled in a turnover process that results from the interplay of degradation from MMPs and the production of matrix components from the fibroblasts.

Pathophysiology of Chronic Wounds

Unlike the orderly healing progression of the acute wound, the chronic wound is stuck in a disorderly mix of inflammation and failed bursts of proliferation. The chronic wound is characterized by four cardinal defects.

■ *Inflammatory excess.* Excessive inflammation occurs, with over-production of inflammatory cytokines, such as IL-6, tumor necrosis factor alpha (TNFα), and MMPs, particularly MMP-1, MMP-8, and MMP-13. This allows altered matrix substances to accumulate, such as fibronectin, which have been rendered ineffectual by protein degradation.

■ *Deficiency of essential growth factors.* Essential growth factors are lacking, in part because of excessive degradation by this hostile wound environment. As a result, cell recruitment, matrix formation, and angiogenesis become impaired.

■ *Bacterial overgrowth and colonization.* Bacteria often congregate in colonies under protective structures called biofilms, which protect them from host defenses. Moreover, the bacteria in their sequestered spaces communicate with small molecules in a process called quorum sensing, and they activate virulence factors. The bacterial cell wall and lipopolysaccharide are capable of activating inflammatory pathways through a toll-like receptor mechanism, which activates nuclear factor-kappaB (NFκB).

■ *Senescence of fibroblasts.* Abnormal aging of fibroblasts makes them less responsive to the stimulatory signals of the healing wound.

Providing good wound care addresses these individual defects, treats the underlying cause (pressure, edema, vasculitis), and reverses the abnormalities, allowing the wound to progress to proliferation with granulation, contraction, re-epithelialization, and scarring—that is, to healing.

The Wound in Diabetes

Chronic wounds differ greatly from acute wounds in the lack of orderly progression to healing, yet they all share the common cardinal defects as listed above. The more difficult question is whether a diabetic foot ulcer is unique as a chronic wound in its pathogenesis and pathophysiology. The following discussion highlights the factors found in the diabetic foot ulcer that distinguish it from other chronic wounds (see Table 1).

Neuropathy

Clearly, the most important factor contributing to the development of foot ulcers and faulty healing is peripheral neuropathy, especially

Table 1. Factors Found in Diabetes and Impaired Wound Healing

Peripheral neuropathy
- Loss of protective sensation
- Autonomic dysfunction
- Impaired neuroinflammatory reflex

Wound hypoxia
- Macrovascular disease
- Microvascular disease
  - Capillary loss
  - Microvascular endothelial dysfunction

Abnormal cellular pathways
- Chemotaxis
- Fibroblast responsiveness

Excess inflammation
- Oxidative stress
- Endothelial dysfunction and impaired nitric oxide signaling
- Increased inflammatory cytokine expression
- Advanced glycosylation end products (AGEs) and receptors (RAGE)

Deficient precursor cells

the loss of protective sensation. Neuropathy permits the recurrent injury sustained in daily walking to build into a crescendo of inflammatory activity that leads to tissue strain and injury, all without detection by the host. The ulceration's initial lesion is a "hot spot" of inflammation over an area of high pressure that is detectable with dermal thermography. Moreover, patients with neuropathy also have limited joint mobility and bony deformities, which contribute to higher plantar foot pressures, thus creating the unfortunate combination of high foot pressures and an inability to feel them. This results in callus formation, more pressure and injury, and ultimately, ulceration (see Chapter 2).

Macrovascular Disease

Part of the faulty healing seen in diabetes can be attributed to wound hypoxia from both macrovascular and microvascular disease. Diabetes is a cardiovascular disease equivalent. In the extremities, people with diabetes are 4 to 5 times more likely to develop peripheral arterial disease (PAD) than are people without diabetes. PAD risk increases even before the onset of hyperglycemia in type 2 diabetes, implicating the prediabetic state in its pathogenesis. This state is characterized by insulin resistance, oxidative stress, and altered free fatty acid (FFA) metabolism. This milieu leads to endothelial dysfunction, with impaired nitric oxide signaling and vasoreactivity, which, through complex mechanisms, result in vasoconstriction, inflammation, and hypercoagulability. These factors may account for the high risk of vascular disease seen in diabetes.

Diabetes is unique as a risk factor not only for its power but also for its predilection to involve the small arteries below the knee, the tibial vessels. Here the disease is typically diffuse and distal, but it spares the arteries of the foot. In addition, PAD is strongly associated with neuropathy, which allows the vascular disease to worsen slowly without sensory feedback. Thus, a patient with diabetes may have severe PAD and ischemia with few or no symptoms and may present late in the course of the disease with an ischemic ulceration.

Microvascular Disease

Patients with diabetes and neuropathy also have significant microvascular defects. Hyperglycemia is associated with a ubiquitous involvement of the microvasculature that is manifested by capillary sclerosis and dropout, particularly in people with type 1 diabetes. This can be seen with capillaroscopy and measurement of elevated capillary pressures. In type 2 patients with neuropathy, functional microvascular abnormalities can be seen, specifically endothelial dysfunction and impaired vasoreactivity. These abnormalities are best demonstrated by laser Doppler imaging of the microcirculation with defective vasodilatory response to heat (generalized defect), acetylcholine (endothelial defect), and sodium nitroprusside (vascular smooth muscle defect). In addition, neuropathy affects the neuroinflammatory microvascular vasodilatation in response to injury or noxious stimuli—the Lewis triple flare.

Impaired angiogenesis is also seen in diabetes. Among many inputs into angiogenesis are neural mediators such as acetylcholine, substance P, and neuropeptide Y—substances involved in the impaired neuroinflammatory response. The presence of peripheral neuropathy may contribute to impaired angiogenesis and wound healing on a cellular basis.

Cellular/Inflammatory Pathways

Diabetes is known to affect the cellular and inflammatory pathways that are involved in wound healing. Hyperglycemia, primarily through a hyperosmotic effect, may slow neutrophil chemotaxis. In vitro studies of fibroblasts taken from subjects with diabetes show altered function and response to stimulatory challenges.

Diabetes is a state of chronic vascular inflammation. A vast body of literature suggests that altered glucose and FFA metabolism results in oxidative stress, endothelial dysfunction, and activation of inflammatory cytokines, in particular those regulated by NFκB. In diabetes, one can demonstrate increased expression of TNFα, TGFβ, IL-6, and other inflammatory factors. These factors are also overexpressed in chronic wounds and probably amplified in the inflammatory milieu of diabetes.

NFκB has several parallel signaling pathways in the skin. Activation may result from physical injury, from toll-like receptors that bind bacterial cell wall components, and from activation by IL-1β and TNFα. In the diabetic foot ulcer, inflammation in the wound is sustained by several pathways that ultimately amplify and augment the response.

In addition, a tonic stimulation of inflammatory signaling is maintained by the accumulation of advanced glycosylation end products (AGEs) and activation of their receptors (RAGE). The RAGE pathway also ultimately activates NFκB. In fact, it has been demonstrated that feeding diabetic mice a high-AGE diet results in impaired wound healing. One can see that the interplay of these separate signaling pathways causes an unfortunate synergy in producing and maintaining inflammation in a nonhealing chronic wound.

Inflammation also leads to increased fibrosis, and the limited joint mobility seen in the diabetic foot probably results from inflammatory excess rather than collagen cross-linking and tendon shortening, as commonly thought.

Finally, new concepts in wound healing and tissue repair highlight the fact that many of the endothelial cells and fibroblasts that repopulate the wound are derived from circulating precursor cells that originate from bone marrow stem cells. This pathway has been shown to be impaired in animal models of diabetes. In addition, patients with diabetes and/or cardiovascular risk factors with endothelial dysfunction have fewer circulating precursor cells than normal control subjects, a fact that may contribute to vascular repair failure and impaired wound healing.

Systemic interventions, in addition to good foot ulcer care, may affect inflammation. Controlling hyperglycemia, oxidative stress, endothelial dysfunction, AGE formation, or other metabolic consequences of diabetes may help reduce inflammatory activity generally and, specifically, its contribution to the excess inflammation seen in diabetic foot ulcers.

Summary

The most common pathway to amputation occurs in people with diabetes and neuropathy who develop a foot ulcer, usually from the recurrent mechanical trauma of daily ambulation. Then faulty healing sets in, ultimately leading to the loss of the limb. Faulty healing is present in all chronic wounds, by definition, and the defect is seen as a lack of progression through the hierarchical stages of healing. The chronic wound is stuck in the inflammatory phase.

Foot ulcers in patients with diabetes differ from other chronic wounds largely by the loss of protective sensation that results from peripheral neuropathy. In addition, limited joint mobility translates into higher foot pressures, which increase the likelihood of mechanical injury.

The faulty healing of diabetes is also a result of wound hypoxia from macrovascular disease. Microvascular disease, both anatomic and physiological, contributes to the abnormal flow, inflammatory response, and angiogenesis seen in patients with diabetes and neuropathy. These factors contribute to impaired healing of foot ulcers.

The cellular responses of neutrophils and fibroblasts that are necessary for healing are also affected by diabetes. Finally, the inflammatory milieu found in diabetes may contribute to and amplify the already heightened inflammation that characterizes all chronic wounds and prevents their normal progression to healing. Systemic interventions could have their greatest impact here, putting the diabetic foot ulcer out of its inflammatory state and into a phase of healthy proliferation and wound healing.

Bibliography

Agren MS, Steenfos HH, Dabelsteen S, Hansen JB, Dabelsteen E: Proliferation and mitogenic response to PDGF-BB of fibroblasts isolated from chronic venous leg ulcers is ulcer-age dependent. *J Invest Dermatol* 112:463–469, 1999

American Diabetes Association: Consensus Development Conference on Diabetic Foot Wound Care: 7–8 April 1999, Boston, Massachusetts. *Diabetes Care* 22: 1354–1360, 1999

American Diabetes Association: Peripheral arterial disease in people with diabetes. *Diabetes Care* 26:3333–3341, 2003

Barone EJ, Yager DR, Pozez AL, Olutoye OO, Crossland MC, Diegelmann RF, Cohen IK: Interleukin-1 alpha and collagenase activity are elevated in chronic wounds. *Plast Reconstr Surg* 102:1023–1027, 1998

Gibran NS, Jang YC, Isik FF, Greenhalgh DG, Muffley LA, Underwood RA, Usui ML, Larsen J, Smith DG, Bunnett N, Ansel JC, Olerud JE: Diminished neuropeptide levels contribute to the impaired cutaneous healing response associated with diabetes mellitus. *J Surg Res* 108:122–128, 2002

Greenberg EP: Bacterial communication and group behavior. *J Clin Invest* 112:1288–1290, 2003

Montesinos MC, Shaw JP, Yee H, Shamamian P, Cronstein BN: Adenosine A(2A) receptor activation promotes wound neovascularization by stimulating angiogenesis and vasculogenesis. *Am J Pathol* 164:1887–1892, 2004

Pecoraro RE, Reiber GE, Burgess EM: Pathways to diabetic limb amputation: basis for prevention. *Diabetes Care* 13:513–521, 1990

Peppa M, Brem H, Ehrlich P, Zhang JG, Cai W, Li Z, Croitoru A, Thung S, Vlassara H: Adverse effects of dietary glycotoxins on wound healing in genetically diabetic mice. *Diabetes* 52:2805–2813, 2003

Robert C, Kupper TS: Inflammatory skin diseases, T cells, and immune surveillance. *N Engl J Med* 341:1817–1828, 1999

Singer AJ, Clark RA: Cutaneous wound healing. *N Engl J Med* 341:738–746, 1999

Steed DL: The role of growth factors in wound healing. *Surg Clin North Am* 77:575–586, 1997

Veves A, Akbari CM, Primavera J, Donaghue VM, Zacharoulis D, Chrzan JS, DeGirolami U, LoGerfo FW, Freeman R: Endothelial dysfunction and the expression of endothelial nitric oxide synthetase in diabetic neuropathy, vascular disease, and foot ulceration. *Diabetes* 47:457–463, 1998

1

Pathogenesis of Diabetic Foot Complications

Andrew J. M. Boulton, MD, DSc (Hon), FRCP

FOOT COMPLICATIONS, which include foot ulceration, neuropathic osteoarthropathy (Charcot foot), and amputation, are common among patients with diabetes. It is estimated that >5% of these patients have a history of foot ulcers, and the cumulative lifetime incidence may be as high as 15%. Some 85% of all amputations are preceded by foot ulcers; therefore, reducing the incidence of foot ulcers should reduce the number of amputations as well (1).

Risk Factors

Foot ulcers rarely result from a single pathology; two or more factors contribute. The neuropathic foot does not spontaneously ulcerate. Insensitivity combined with either extrinsic factors (such as walking barefoot and stepping on a sharp object or simply wearing ill-fitting shoes) or intrinsic factors (a patient with insensitivity and callus walks and develops an ulcer) ultimately results in ulceration. Neuropathy is the most important cause of ulceration.

Neuropathy

The association between both somatic and autonomic neuropathy and foot ulceration has long been recognized, but only in the last decade have prospective follow-up studies confirmed the role of somatic neuropathy in causing foot ulcers. Patients with sensory loss appear to have up to a sevenfold increased risk of developing foot ulcers, compared with nonneuropathic diabetic individuals (2). Poor balance and instability are increasingly being recognized as troublesome symptoms of peripheral neuropathy, presumably secondary to proprioceptive loss.

Peripheral autonomic (sympathetic) dysfunction results in dry skin and, in the absence of peripheral arterial disease, a warm foot with distended dorsal foot veins. However, because patients often think that all foot problems result from vascular disease, some may find it difficult to accept that their warm but pain-free feet are at significant risk of unperceived trauma and subsequent ulceration.

In practice, peripheral neuropathy can easily be determined by examining the foot for evidence of neuropathy—detailed quantitative sensory testing or electrophysiology is not needed. Simple tools such as a modified neuropathy disability score (2) and the monofilament may be used to help identify the at-risk neuropathic foot. (Additional details about the foot exam are provided in Chapter 2.)

Peripheral Arterial Disease

In approximately a third of all cases, peripheral ischemia resulting from proximal arterial disease is a contributing factor in ulceration. The ischemic foot is red, dry, and often neuropathic, so it is susceptible to pressure from footwear, for example.

Other Risk Factors

The presence of foot deformity, particularly claw toes and prominent metatarsal heads, is a proven risk factor for ulceration. Similarly, one cross-sectional study (3) showed that plantar callus accumulation was associated with an 11-fold increase in risk. In follow-up with these patients, plantar ulcers occurred only at sites of callus in neuropathic feet. Other risk factors include the presence of other microvascular complications, long duration of diabetes, increases in plantar foot pressures, and peripheral edema. Most predictive of all was a past history of foot ulcers or amputation.

Prevention

Education

Preventing foot ulcers among those with risk factors is key to reducing the incidence of ulcers. Unfortunately, studies of preventive education have not confirmed its usefulness. Education along with regular podiatric care, however, may result in earlier presentation when ulcers develop.

A few studies have assessed psychosocial factors (4). Patients' behavior is apparently not driven by being designated "at risk"— rather, it is driven by the patients' own perception of their risks. Thus, if patients believe that a foot ulcer could lead to amputation, they are more likely to follow educational advice on how to reduce ulcer risk. Figure 1.1 outlines a pathway to foot ulceration, including areas where psychosocial factors are relevant. Additional research in this area is urgently required.

Foot Examinations

The most important aspect of diagnosing the foot at risk of ulceration is regularly asking patients to remove their shoes and socks and examining the foot in detail for evidence of neuropathy, vascular disease, deformities, plantar callus, edema, and other risk factors. A simple foot pressure mat (such as the PressureStat system; Foot Logic, New York) can help identify high pressures under the diabetic foot. Furthermore, these pressure maps of the foot, which show higher pressure areas as darker, may be used to educate patients about their risk for subsequent ulceration.

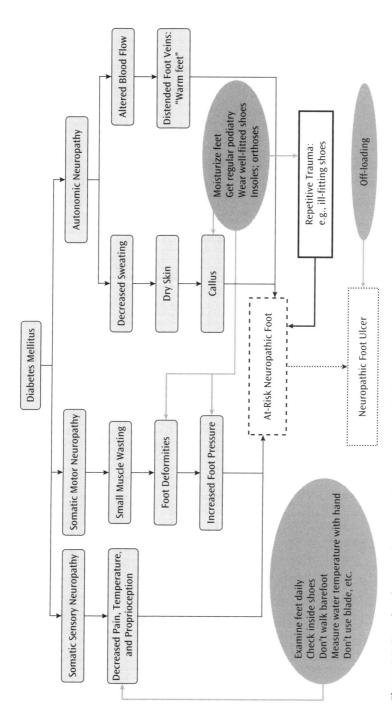

Figure 1.1 Causal pathways to foot ulceration, emphasizing the key role of the patient in ulcer prevention (spheres). *From* Boulton, reprinted with permission.

The Pathway to Ulceration

The combination of two or more of the risks factors discussed above ultimately results in diabetic foot ulceration. Various work (5–7) has suggested that the most common triad leading to breakdown of the diabetic foot includes peripheral neuropathy (insensitivity), deformity (clawing of the toes, prominence of metatarsal heads), and trauma (from footwear and/or repetitive stress). Other simple examples of a two-component pathway to ulceration are neuropathy and mechanical trauma (such as standing on a nail) or neuropathy and thermal trauma (inappropriate use of chemical "corn cures" or when a patient with insensate feet uses a heating pack).

The Patient with Sensory Loss

To reduce neuropathic foot problems, keep in mind that patients with insensitivity have lost the warning signal—pain—that ordinarily brings the patient to their doctor. Pain often leads to medical consultations, and our training and health care focus on the cause and relief of symptoms. Thus, the care of the patient with no pain sensation is a challenge for which we have little training. However, we can learn from those who treat leprosy, another disease in which patients' loss of pain diminishes their motivation to heal and prevent injury.

Charcot Neuroarthropathy

Charcot neuroarthropathy (CN) occurs in patients with peripheral loss of sensation and autonomic dysfunction (increased blood flow to the foot and dry skin), usually with unperceived trauma. The patient at risk of CN typically has a warm foot with bounding pulses but complete loss of sensation. Any patient presenting with unilateral warm, swollen foot, with or without symptoms of pain or discomfort, and good circulation should be considered to have Charcot neuroarthropathy until proven otherwise. (Chapter 9 discusses the presentation and management of CN.)

References

1. Singh N, Armstrong DG, Lipsky BA: Preventing foot ulcers in persons with diabetes. *JAMA.* In press

2. Abbott CA, Carrington AL, Ashe H, Bath S, Every LC, Griffiths J, Hann AW, Hussein A, Jackson N, Johnson KE, Ryder CH, Torkington R, Van Ross ER, Whalley AM, Widdows P, Williamson S, Boulton AJ: The North-West Diabetes Foot Care Study: Incidence of, and risk factors for, new diabetic foot ulceration in a community-based patient cohort. *Diabet Med* 19:377–384, 2002

3. Murray HJ, Young MJ, Hollis S, Boulton AJ: The association between callus formation, high pressures and neuropathy in diabetic foot ulceration. *Diabetic Med* 13:979–982, 1996

4. Vileikyte L, Rubin RR, Leventhal H: Psychological aspects of diabetic neuropathic foot complications: an overview. *Diabetes Metab Res Rev* 20 (Suppl. 1):S13–S18, 2004

5. Lavery LA, Armstrong DG, Vela SA, Quebedeaux TL, Fleischli JG: Practical criteria for screening patients at high risk for diabetic foot ulceration. *Arch Intern Med* 158:157–162, 1998

6. Reiber GE, Vileikyte L, Boyko EJ, del Aguila M, Smith DG, Lavery LA, Boulton AJ: Causal pathways for incident lower-extremity ulcers in patients with diabetes from two settings. *Diabetes Care* 22:157–162, 1999

7. Armstrong DG, Lavery LA, Nixon BP, Boulton AJM: It's not what you put on, but what you take off: techniques for debriding and off-loading the diabetic foot wound. *Clin Infect Dis* 39 (Suppl. 2):S92–S99, 2004

Bibliography

Boulton AJM: *The Diabetic Foot—From Art to Science: 18th Camillo Golgi Lecture.* Reference 04/274. Bristol, UK, Springer-Verlag GmbH, 2004

Boulton AJM, Kirsner RS, Vileikyte L: Neuropathic diabetic foot ulcers. *N Engl J Med* 351:48–55, 2004

Brem H, Sheehan P, Boulton AJ: Protocol for treatment of diabetic foot ulcers. *Am J Surg* 187 (Suppl. 5a):1S–10S, 2004

Jeffcoate WJ, Harding KG: Diabetic foot ulcers. *Lancet* 361:1545–1551, 2003

Van Houtum WH, Bakker K (Eds.): The diabetic foot: proceedings of the 4th international symposium on the diabetic foot. *Diabet Metab Res Rev* 20 (Suppl.): S1–S95, 2004

2

The Diabetic Foot Examination

Nalini Singh, MD
John Giurini, DPM

EXAMINING THE DIABETIC FOOT is essential to preventing ulcers and amputations. Incorporating a thorough foot examination into a busy primary care practice may seem challenging, but a few simple interventions can improve provider compliance and efficiency. These include clinical reminders in the patient's medical chart and algorithms for interventions and referral based on risk stratification (1–3). Asking patients to remove their shoes when they enter the examining room facilitates the process (2–4), and nurses can learn to perform foot screenings and report worrisome findings to the primary care provider. Finally, patients themselves can be instructed to remind their providers about the foot examination and to seek medical attention when foot problems arise (5).

Patient History/Risk Factors

The purpose of foot examinations is to identify individuals at risk for foot ulceration and amputation. (See Table 2.1 for an overview of the diabetic foot examination.) Before performing the exam, the health

Table 2.1 The Diabetic Foot Examination

Assessment	Tests	Significant Findings
Patient history		• Previous foot ulceration • Previous amputation • Diabetes >10 yr • A1C ≥7% • Impaired vision • Neuropathic symptoms • Claudication
Gross inspection		• Corns, calluses, bunions • Prominent metatarsal heads • Hammertoes, claw toes
Dermatologic examination		• Dry skin • Absence of hair • Yellow or erythematous scales • Yellow, thickened nails • Ingrown nail edges, long or sharp nails • Interspace maceration • Ulceration
Screening for neuropathy	• Semmes-Weinstein monofilament (10 g) • Vibration perception threshold testing • Tuning fork (128 Hz)	• Lack of perception at one or more sites • Abnormal perception of vibration • Vibration perception threshold >25 volts

Table 2.1 The Diabetic Foot Examination (*continued*)

Assessment	Tests	Significant Findings
Vascular examination	• Palpation of dorsalis pedis and posterior tibial pulses • Ankle-brachial index (ABI)	• Absent pulses • ABI <0.90, consistent with peripheral arterial disease
Biomechanical foot assessment	• Plantarflexion/dorsiflexion of ankles and great toes • Watching patient ambulate • Inspection of patient's shoes • Assessment of patient's ability to see and reach his or her feet	• Diminished joint mobility • Decreased vision, gait imbalance, need for assistive devices • Ill-fitting footwear • Patient's inability to see and reach his or her feet

care provider should ask the patient about diabetes-specific risk factors (6,7), such as

■ previous foot ulcerations or amputation
■ duration of diabetes >10 years
■ suboptimal glycemic control (A1C ≥7%)
■ impaired vision

The provider should also inquire about

■ previous foot problems or surgery
■ neuropathic foot symptoms such as numbness; tingling; hot or cold sensations; and aching, burning or lancinating pain
■ hyperesthesia (8,9)
■ leg claudication (8,9)

Gross Inspection

During the foot exam, the patient should be sitting barefoot with his or her legs extended (10). Gross inspection may reveal corns, calluses, and common foot deformities, such as bunions, prominent metatarsal heads, and hammertoes or claw toes, which increase plantar pressures and contribute to foot ulcerations (10–12).

Dermatologic Examination

Inspect the patient's skin—dry skin can crack and form fissures that serve as potential portals of entry for infection (13). Shiny, hairless skin can be a sign of peripheral arterial disease. Yellow or erythematous scales could indicate tinea pedis, and yellow, thickened nails could signal onychomycosis. Treating fungal foot infections reduces the incidence of lower-extremity cellulitis (14,15). Check between the patient's toes for maceration and moisture; patients are often unaware that these areas are especially vulnerable to skin breakdown. The provider should also point out any ingrown nail edges and very long or sharp nails, which could lacerate adjacent toes. Any foot ulceration warrants an urgent referral to a podiatrist or wound care specialist (16–21).

Screening Tools

Semmes-Weinstein Monofilament

In primary care, the Semmes-Weinstein monofilament (SWM) is the most widely used proven tool to screen for sensory peripheral neuropathy (22). This quick and inexpensive test consists of a rod with a nylon filament that buckles into a C shape with the application of 10 grams of force (22). The SWM is applied at 10 sites—the plantar surfaces of the first, third, and fifth digits and metatarsal heads, the plantar midfoot medially and laterally, the plantar heel, and the dorsal first web space (Fig. 2.1; 22–25). With the patient's eyes closed, the provider applies the SWM and asks the patient to identify the cor-

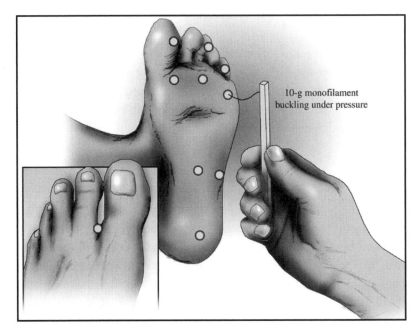

Figure 2.1 Application of the Semmes-Weinstein monofilament to 10 sites on the foot. Artist: Chris Pacheco, VA Puget Sound

rect foot and location. Lack of perception of the SWM at one or more sites is associated with clinically significant large-fiber neuropathy (22) and identifies the patient as at risk for ulceration. Note: After being used on >10 patients/day, the SWM loses its accuracy and requires a recovery period of 24 h (26).

Tuning Forks and Biothesiometers

The provider should test for vibratory perception with the tuning fork, or if available, the biothesiometer. A vibrating 128-Hz tuning fork is placed on the dorsal interphalangeal joint of the great toe, and the patient is instructed to report when the vibration ceases (27). The provider may place the index finger of his or her free hand in the sulcus under the patient's toe to monitor the accuracy of the patient's perception. The biothesiometer consists of a handheld device with a rubber tactor that vibrates at 100–120 Hz. A stylus is placed on the tip of the great toe, perpendicular to the surface. While the examiner increases the voltage with the dial, the patient reports when he or she perceives the vibration. A vibration perception threshold (VPT) >25 volts indicates a sensory deficit. The combination of either decreased SWM perception or a VPT >25 volts yields 100% sensitivity and 77% specificity for predicting foot ulceration (25).

Vascular Examination

The examiner should attempt to palpate the dorsalis pedis and posterior tibial pulses. The dorsalis pedis may be palpated most easily with the examiner's second and third finger pads when the patient dorsiflexes the foot. The posterior tibial pulse is best detected when the foot is inverted (10). If it is difficult to palpate the pulses, a hand-held Doppler ultrasound can help. The accuracy of pedal pulses may vary with the examiner's experience. Experts recommend the ankle-brachial index (ABI) to diagnose peripheral arterial disease, as it is 95% sensitive and almost 100% specific when compared to vascular disease proven by angiography (28).

With the hand-held Doppler device, measure the systolic blood pressure in the dorsalis pedis and posterior tibial arteries and the brachial arteries, and calculate the ratio. An ABI of <0.90 indicates peripheral arterial disease, with the ABI scores interpreted as follows (28):

- 0.70–0.90: mild PAD
- 0.40–0.69: moderate PAD
- <0.40: severe PAD

Note that with medial artery calcinosis and diabetes, however, the ABI will be falsely elevated and does not reliably predict the severity of vascular disease (13). In these cases, other methods are more accurate, e.g., toe blood pressure, transcutaneous oxygen pressures, Doppler arterial waveforms (28–30).

Biomechanical Foot Assessment

Because decreased joint mobility has been shown to increase plantar pressure and foot ulcer risk, the provider should perform a biomechanical foot assessment (31). The patient should be asked to plantarflex and dorsiflex his or her ankle joint maximally (10). Normal gait requires that a person be able to dorsiflex the great toe 45–50 degrees and plantarflex 10 degrees. Watching the patient walk allows the provider to assess the patient's risk for foot complications and note vision, balance, and need for assistive devices. In addition, inspect the patient's shoes to ensure that they fit comfortably. They should be wide enough to accommodate the span of the foot at the metatarsophalangeal joints.

The examiner should also assess whether the patient can see and reach both the top and bottom of his or her feet, because one study showed that up to 80% of elderly patients cannot see or reach their feet (32). If the patient cannot do this, he or she could use special equipment, such as a long-handled mirror or brush with sponges to reach between the toes. In addition, a family member or caregiver should be taught how to inspect and care for the patient's feet.

Summary

At the end of the examination, document all findings and assign the patient to a risk category using the risk classification system proposed by the International Working Group on the Diabetic Foot (19) in 1999 (see also Table 3.1, page 33). An annual examination suffices for patients in the 0 risk category, because they are at low risk for ulceration. A patient with mild sensory neuropathy (category 1) should have a foot examination every six months; patients in the highest risk categories (2 and 3) should visit a foot specialist at least every three months and more frequently if they have acute problems (7,33).

Various interventions are appropriate for patients in each risk category: education, special footwear, referrals to foot specialists, and more frequent foot examinations by the provider.

References

1. Khoury A, Landers P, Roth M, Rowe N, DaMert G, Dahar W, Nystrom H, Szczepanik R: Computer-supported identification and intervention for diabetic patients at risk for amputation. *MD Comput* 15:307–310, 1998

2. Wylie-Rosett J, Walker EA, Shamoon H, Engel S, Basch C, Zybert P: Assessment of documented foot examinations for patients with diabetes in inner-city primary care clinics. *Arch Fam Med* 4:46–50, 1995

3. O'Brien KE, Chandramohan V, Nelson DA, Fischer JR, Stevens G, Poremba JA: Effect of a physician-directed educational campaign on performance of proper diabetic foot exams in an outpatient setting. *J Gen Intern Med* 18:258–265, 2003

4. Bailey TS, Yu HM, Rayfield E: Patterns of foot examination in a diabetes clinic. *Am J Med* 78:371–374, 1985

5. Williams JA: We make foot exams a priority. *RN* 64:40–41, 2001

6. Boyko EJ, Ahroni JH, Stensel V, Forsberg RC, Davignon DR, Smith DG: A prospective study of risk factors for diabetic foot ulcer. The Seattle Diabetic Foot Study. *Diabetes Care* 22:1036–1042, 1999

7. Lavery LA, Armstrong DG, Vela SA, Quebedeaux TL, Fleischli JG: Practical criteria for screening patients at high risk for diabetic foot ulceration. *Arch Intern Med* 158:157–162, 1998

8. Boulton AJ: Guidelines for diagnosis and outpatient management of diabetic peripheral neuropathy. European Association for the Study of Diabetes, Neurodiab. *Diabetes Metab* 24 (Suppl. 3):55–65, 1998

9. Mayfield JA, Reiber GE, Sanders LJ, Janisse D, Pogach LM: Preventive foot care in people with diabetes. *Diabetes Care* 21:2161–2177, 1998

10. Altman MI, Altman KS: The podiatric assessment of the diabetic lower extremity: special considerations. *Wounds* 12 (Suppl. B):64B–71B, 2000

11. Boulton AJM, Vileikyte L: Pathogenesis of diabetic foot ulceration and measurements of neuropathy. *Wounds* 12 (Suppl. B):12B–18B, 2000

12. Boike AM, Hall JO: A practical guide for examining and treating the diabetic foot. *Cleve Clin J Med* 69:342–348, 2002

13. Rosenblum BI: Identifying the patient at risk of foot ulceration. *Wounds* 12 (Suppl. B):7B–11B, 2000

14. Baddour LM, Bisno AL: Recurrent cellulitis after coronary bypass surgery: association with superficial fungal infection in saphenous venectomy limbs. *JAMA* 251:1049–1052, 1984

15. Karakas M, Baba M, Aksungur VL, Memisoglu HR, Aksungur EH, Denli YG, Karakas P: Manifestation of cellulitis after saphenous venectomy for coronary bypass surgery. *J Eur Acad Dermatol Venereol* 16:438–440, 2002

16. American Diabetes Association: Preventative foot care in people with diabetes (Position Statement). *Diabetes Care* 27 (Suppl. 1):S63–S64, 2004

17. Hutchinson A, McIntosh A, Feder G, Home PD, Young R: *Clinical Guideline for Type 2 Diabetes: Prevention and Management of Foot Problems.* London, Royal College of General Practitioners, 2000

18. Veterans Health Administration/Department of Defense Office of Quality and Performance: *Clinical Practice Guidelines: Diabetes Mellitus Algorithms. Module F: Foot Care,* 1999

19. International Working Group on the Diabetic Foot: *International Consensus on the Diabetic Foot.* Amsterdam, Netherlands, International Diabetes Federation, 2003

20. Wheatley C: Audit protocol: Part one: Prevention of diabetic foot ulcers: the noncomplicated foot. *J Clin Govern* 9:93–100, 2001

21. Wheatley C, Shaw C: Audit protocol: Part two: Management of diabetic foot ulcers: the 'at risk' foot. *J Clin Govern* 9:157–162, 2001

22. Armstrong DG: The 10-g monofilament: the diagnostic divining rod for the diabetic foot? [Editorial]. *Diabetes Care* 23:887, 2000

23. Mayfield JA, Sugarman JR: The use of the Semmes-Weinstein monofilament and other threshold tests for preventing foot ulceration and amputation in persons with diabetes. *J Fam Pract* 49:S17–S29, 2000

24. Armstrong DG: Loss of protective sensation: a practical evidence-based definition. *J Foot Ankle Surg* 38:79–80, 1999

25. Armstrong DG, Lavery LA, Vela SA, Quebedeaux TL, Fleischli JG: Choosing a practical screening instrument to identify patients at risk for diabetic foot ulceration. *Arch Intern Med* 158:289–292, 1998

26. Booth J, Young MJ: Differences in the performance of commercially available 10-g monofilaments. *Diabetes Care* 23:984–988, 2000

27. Liniger C, Albeanu A, Bloise D, Assal JP: The tuning fork revisited. *Diabet Med* 7:859–864, 1990

28. American Diabetes Association: Peripheral arterial disease in people with diabetes (Position Statement). *Diabetes Care* 26:3333–3341, 2003

29. Vowden P: Doppler ultrasound in the management of the diabetic foot. *The Diabetic Foot* 2 (Suppl.):16–17, 1999

30. Sykes MT, Godsey JB: Vascular evaluation of the problem diabetic foot. *Clin Podiatr Med Surg* 15:49–83, 1998

31. Lavery L, Gazewood JD: Assessing the feet of patients with diabetes. *J Fam Pract* 49:S9–S16, 2000

32. Thomson FJ, Masson EA: Can elderly diabetic patients cooperate with routine foot care? *Age Ageing* 21:333–337, 1992

33. Peters EJ, Lavery LA, International Working Group on the Diabetic Foot: Effectiveness of the diabetic foot risk classification system of the International Working Group on the Diabetic Foot. *Diabetes Care* 24:1442–1447, 2001

3

Foot Risk Classification and Prevention

Edgar J. G. Peters, MD, PhD
Karel Bakker, MD, PhD

T WO SIGNIFICANT COMPLICATIONS of diabetes are foot ulcers and lower-extremity amputations. Amputations by themselves have been associated with an increased risk of recurrent ulceration and additional amputations, as well as a high incidence of mortality and morbidity. Several risk factors associated with the development of foot complications are peripheral symmetric neuropathy, vascular impairment, limited joint mobility, foot deformities, ill-fitting footwear, penetrating trauma, and abnormal foot pressures on the sole of the foot (1,2). Severe hyperglycemia is related to the occurrence of risk factors and subsequent complications.

Initiatives such as Healthy People 2010 seek to prevent as much as 55% of amputations in patients with diabetes. This reduction can be achieved by adequate screening for risk factors, treatment in multispecialty diabetic foot teams, and optimal prevention. Regretfully, in many medical facilities, systematic foot screenings to identify patients with risk factors for diabetic foot complications are simply not performed.

Risk Factors

Peripheral Neuropathy

Distal symmetric peripheral neuropathy is one of the strongest risk factors for foot complications in patients with diabetes mellitus (1). With nerve damage, the patient might complain of loss of sensation, numbness, or difficulty maintaining balance. Involvement of the motor nerves can lead to muscle atrophy, alteration of muscle balance, and thus to flexion deformities (claw toes) and increased pressure on the metatarsal heads and dorsal aspect of the toes. Autonomic neuropathy can cause dry skin by diminished transpiration and arteriovenous shunting.

Nerve function can be tested in several ways, some of which are technically difficult or cumbersome. For screening situations it is more convenient to identify patients by using simple, bedside-applicable techniques (2). Semmes-Weinstein monofilaments, vibration perception threshold (VPT), or a combination of these modalities can be used to identify patients at risk for foot ulceration. (Methods to assess loss of protective sensation are discussed in further detail in Chapter 2.) So far, only intensive glucose control has proved effective in preserving sensory nerve function (3).

Arterial Disease

Peripheral arterial disease (PAD) is common in patients with diabetes and is one of the causes of diabetic foot problems (1,2). PAD contributes to faulty wound healing and subsequent amputation. Arterial disease is likely an important risk factor for foot ulceration, and some studies have indeed linked arterial impairment to the development of diabetic foot ulcers (1). (Diabetic foot specialists usually distinguish between ischemic ulcers and neuropathic ulcers.) However, recent reports have denied a significant univariate or multivariate association between either micro- or macrovascular disease and development of an ulcer.

In this respect, arterial disease could be more a risk factor for the failure of ulcers to heal and thus for amputation than a direct risk factor for the ulceration itself. Whatever its exact role, peripheral arterial disease remains a critically important consideration in any focused physical examination.

Important ways to screen for vascular problems are by palpation of peripheral arteries, ankle-brachial index (ABI), and transcutaneous oxygen pressure (tcPO$_2$). A low ABI—that is, <0.9—indicates arterial disease. Although an ABI can sometimes give unrealistically high results in the presence of calcified vessels (medial or Mönckeberg's calcinosis), it is a valuable clinical instrument. Toe systolic pressure is more precise, but the technique is time consuming and more expensive. Transcutaneous oxygen pressure measures the partial oxygen pressure at the skin surface. Patients with values >30 mmHg usually do not have critical limb ischemia, but tcPO$_2$ is variable under local vasodilatory or vasoconstrictive conditions, such as foot position or edema. More invasive or technically advanced measurements can give more precise indications of the vascular status.

Therapeutic interventions to prevent both cardiac and peripheral arterial disease include correcting lipemia and hypertension, reducing hyperglycemia, and stopping smoking.

Deformity

Either intrinsic foot deformities or a previous amputation can cause deformity in the diabetic foot. In the first case, soft tissue glycosylation is thought to cause joints to stiffen (limited joint mobility) and cushioning footpads to diminish. Another important factor in the development of deformity and high plantar pressure is motor neuropathy. Amputations can lead to abnormal pressures on diverse parts of the foot too, causing additional ulceration and amputations. Areas of abnormal high pressure can be measured using various devices, either platform or in-shoe systems.

Many interventions are directed at reducing peak foot pressure, removing callus on the sole of the foot, and accommodating foot deformities in order to reduce pressure. Simply advising patients to wear appropriate shoe gear, regardless of other risk factors, results in a significant reduction in lower-extremity ulcers. Some researchers advocate elective surgery to correct foot deformities in diabetic patients to heal or prevent diabetic foot ulcers. Procedures such as correction of toe deformity, resectional arthroplasty of the interphalangeal joint, and Achilles tendon lengthening have shown mixed results.

Shoe Gear

Education for both health care providers and patients is a cornerstone in prevention. Ulcers that develop on the dorsum of the toes or over bony prominences on the medial or lateral aspect of the foot and that are not otherwise attributable to direct trauma or injury are probably caused by ill-fitting shoes. Preventive measures include wearing shoes that fit properly and perhaps padded hosiery. Most patients do not need to buy traditional therapeutic shoes.

Puncture Injuries

Previous studies have indicated that diabetic patients with puncture injuries and subsequent ulcers were up to 46 times more likely to have an amputation than patients without diabetes. These barefoot puncture injuries are more than twice as common in diabetic patients than in patients without diabetes. However, most objects would not have been able to penetrate if shoes had been worn (4). Again, simple preventive measures and patient education are very effective in reducing injury.

Risk Classification

Patients need to be classified into risk groups so that those at greatest risk get the care they need. Several risk classification systems have been developed over time, some of which used general medical parameters, such as the presence of retinopathy or the patient's level of glycemic control. Some systems were based on more specific (local) risk factors for diabetic foot complications. Only a few studies have been validated with clinical data to predict outcome.

Mayfield et al. (5) validated their classification for amputations, Lavery et al. (1) for ulcerations, and Rith-Najarian et al. (6) and the International Working Group on the Diabetic Foot (IWGDF; 2,7) for both ulcers and amputations. The consensus classification system differs from earlier ones in that clinicians and researchers from various parts of the world and from different specialties were involved in creating it.

IWGDF Consensus Classification

The IWGDF classification was validated with clinical data in a study. Based on risk factors present upon enrollment, subjects were put into four risk groups according to the consensus classification. Group 0 consisted of subjects without sensory neuropathy, group 1 consisted of patients with neuropathy but without deformity or peripheral arterial disease, group 2 consisted of subjects with neuropathy and peripheral arterial disease and/or deformity, and group 3 consisted of patients with a history of foot ulceration or a lower-extremity amputation. The groups, method for categorization, and advised check-up frequency are shown in Table 3.1.

In the study, the higher risk groups had significantly more ulcerations and amputations, as well as a higher proportion of proximal amputations. In fact, patients in the high-risk group are 34 times more likely to ulcerate than patients in the lowest risk group. Likewise, high-risk patients are 17 times more likely to receive an amputation in a three-year follow-up than patients in a lower-risk group. Patients with a history of amputation were shown to be at even greater risk (7).

The objective of the consensus classification was to evaluate patients with diabetes to classify them into risk groups that would predict morbid outcomes. Evaluation tools had to be inexpensive and readily available worldwide so that even the busiest of clinical practices could incorporate them. In addition, the patient's risk classification for diabetic foot complications determines frequency of follow-up. Resources such as therapeutic shoes, education, and clinical visits can then be allocated to patients at greatest risk of adverse

Table 3.1 IWGDF Risk Classification System for Diabetic Foot Complications

	IWGDF Risk Classification System (2,7)	
Category	Risk Profile	Check-up Frequency
0	• No unnoticed pinprick with the Semmes-Weinstein monofilament and/or • Vibration perception threshold <25 volts	Once a year
1	• One or more unnoticed pinpricks with the Semmes-Weinstein monofilament and/or a vibration perception threshold >25 volts • Ankle-brachial index >0.8 and all pedal pulsations palpable • No hallux valgus, rigid toe contractures (such as hammer- or claw toes) or prominent metatarsal heads	Once every 6 mo
2	• One or more unnoticed pinpricks with the Semmes-Weinstein monofilament or a vibration perception threshold >25 volts • Ankle brachial index <0.8 or any pedal pulsation that is not palpable **or** • Hallux valgus, rigid toe contractures (such as hammer- or claw toes), or prominent metatarsal heads	Once every 3 mo
3	• Previous ulcer or amputation	Once every 1–3 mo

events, and a shift from therapeutic medical and surgical treatment to preventive measures might occur (2).

Multidisciplinary Approach

Evidence suggests that clinical management of patients with diabetes mellitus needs a multidisciplinary approach. Each specialist involved in the patient's care should use the same set of definitions and operational variables to facilitate communication. Ideally, patients are treated by a diabetic foot team. Such a foot team should consist of an orthopedic surgeon, a podiatrist (or podiatric surgeon), a vascular surgeon, a diabetologist or internist, an orthopedic shoemaker, and a rehabilitation physician. These specialists can comment on the complex problems of patients with diabetic foot complications based on their specific background.

Summary

The most important risk factors for diabetic foot complications are peripheral symmetric neuropathy, vascular impairment, limited joint mobility, foot deformities, callus, ill-fitting footwear, penetrating trauma, abnormal plantar pressures, and previous foot problems, such as ulcers or amputations. Screening for these risk factors, treatment in multispecialty diabetic foot teams, and optimal prevention will help reduce the number of amputations. Assigning risk is an essential part of the process, and by using the risk classification of the IWGDF, we can determine frequency of check-ups based on risk.

References

1. Lavery LA, Armstrong DG, Vela SA, Quebedeaux TL, Fleischli JG: Practical criteria for screening patients at high risk for diabetic foot ulceration. *Arch Intern Med* 158:157–162, 1998

2. International Working Group on the Diabetic Foot: *International Consensus on the Diabetic Foot.* Amsterdam, Netherlands, International Diabetes Federation, 1999, p. 96. Web site: http://www.iwgdf.org/

3. Reichard P, Nilsson BY, Rosenqvist U: The effect of long-term intensified insulin treatment on the development of microvascular complications of diabetes mellitus. *N Engl J Med* 329:304–309, 1993

4. Lavery LA, Walker SC, Harkless LB, Felder-Johnson K: Infected puncture wounds in diabetic and nondiabetic adults. *Diabetes Care* 18:1588–1591, 1995

5. Mayfield JA, Reiber GE, Nelson RG, Greene T: A foot risk classification system to predict diabetic amputation in Pima Indians. *Diabetes Care* 19:704–709, 1996

6. Rith-Najarian SJ, Stolusky T, Gohdes DM: Identifying diabetic patients at high risk for lower-extremity amputation in a primary health care setting. *Diabetes Care* 15:1386–1389, 1992

7. Peters EJ, Lavery LA: Effectiveness of the diabetic foot risk classification system of the International Working Group on the Diabetic Foot. *Diabetes Care* 24: 1442–1447, 2001

4

Shoes and Insoles for At-Risk People with Diabetes

Jan S. Ulbrecht, MD
Peter R. Cavanagh, PhD, DSc

DIABETES IS THE LEADING CAUSE of nontraumatic lower-extremity amputation, which is usually preceded by a foot ulcer. More than 15% of all people with diabetes will experience a foot ulcer at some point in their lifetime (1). Footwear can both cause and prevent foot injury. Therefore, practitioners treating patients with diabetes must understand the principles and practice of comprehensive foot care, including the prescription of appropriate footwear. The clinician's evaluation of footwear and insoles should be a standard part of the lower-extremity examination.

Who Is at Risk?

As discussed in more detail in Chapter 3, identification of patients at risk for foot injury who will benefit from enhanced self-care and therapeutic footwear begins with an assessment of sensation in the foot. If patients cannot feel the touch of a 10-g monofilament, they are said to have lost protective sensation and thus may injure their feet without knowing it. In patients with foot deformities (such as a prominent metatarsal head, clawed toes, or a midfoot prominence), injury may occur at the site of the deformity because of repetitive elevated plantar pressure during walking. Impaired lower-extremity circulation (indicated, for example, by a low ankle-brachial index [2]) is also a risk factor for foot injury. In addition, all patients with a prior ulcer should be considered at risk, as should patients with any foot amputation, including partial amputation of toes. The risk is greater for those who are more active, because of the increased cumulative stress on the foot.

Evidence Base for Therapeutic Footwear

Footwear as a Cause of Injury

Considerable anecdotal evidence and opinion indicate that shoes can cause foot injury (3–7). Various authors have suggested that 21–82% of foot ulcers are related to pressure from footwear or to narrow or otherwise inadequate footwear. These rates refer primarily to injuries to the dorsal surface of the foot.

Footwear for Primary Prevention

Most foot ulcers occur on the plantar surface at points of high plantar pressure, most frequently under the metatarsal heads. Therapeutic footwear can prevent such ulcers by reducing loading at these points. No studies have yet appeared in the literature that examine the role of footwear in preventing the first ulcer in at-risk people with diabetes. However, footwear can have a protective effect in these individuals, and prescribing appropriate footwear for all patients who have risk factors for foot injury is a prudent measure.

Footwear for Secondary Prevention

Ulcer recurrence is the dominant problem in treating diabetic foot disease. Estimates for recurrence vary from 28% at 12 months (8) to 100% at 40 months (9), and the relative risk of an ulcer for patients with a history of prior ulcer is 57 times that of patients without such history (10). Although it is widely believed that therapeutic footwear can prevent ulcer recurrence, evidence in support of a protective effect comes mainly from clinical studies that were not always randomized or appropriately controlled (8,11–13). Two studies have shown no effect of footwear (14,15), but both these trials had significant design flaws. In the absence of strong evidence, providers of diabetes care should be guided by the prevailing clinical practice of giving patients with healed foot ulcers carefully prescribed therapeutic footwear as part of an overall enhanced foot care program.

Footwear for Patients with Ulcers

Patients with foot ulcers should not wear shoes, because shoes cannot in general provide the mechanical off-loading needed to accomplish healing. Various approaches to off-loading during healing are discussed in Chapter 6.

Practice

The Goals of Footwear Intervention

Therapeutic footwear aims to protect the foot from external injury, reduce pressure on the plantar surface, accommodate dorsal deformity, and provide stability during activities of daily life. Although the provider of diabetes care does not typically have the skills to design therapeutic footwear, he or she should nevertheless understand these goals as a basis for developing a relationship with a local footwear supplier to whom patients can then be referred with confidence.

Most footwear intervention focuses on reducing plantar pressure at regions of high risk, such as the metatarsal heads, tips of clawed toes, and prominences due to bony deformity. In general, this treatment uses thick compliant insoles to provide load relief at high pressure areas, as well as specifically placed "reliefs" or supports (the best known is a metatarsal pad or bar) that transfer load to other regions of the foot. Pedorthists (practitioners who are certified by the Pedorthic

Footwear Association) are skilled in making such modifications, although the scientific basis for effective load-relief techniques is still being developed.

Choice of Footwear

Practitioners prescribing footwear for at-risk patients must consider the lifestyle of the patient. Typically, patients need footwear that is suited to their occupation, leisure activities, and home use, including nighttime barefoot walking that might present a significant risk of ulceration. Table 4.1 presents a guide to prescription footwear based on the patient's activity level and risk of foot injury.

Patients at the low end of the at-risk spectrum can frequently use wide, well-fitting athletic shoes without any modification. Such shoes can reduce plantar pressure by up to 30% and have been reported to reduce plantar callus (16,17). Patients who need more protection should be fitted with "depth shoes," which provide enough height in the forefoot area to allow for a thick insole (flat or customized; see below) without forcing the dorsum of the foot up against the shoe upper.

For patients at high risk, shoes should have rigid "rocker" or "roller" outsoles that, along with an appropriate insole, allow patients to walk without significantly extending their toes at the metatarsophalangeal joints. This design has been shown to reduce plantar pressure by as much as 50% (18). A qualified pedorthist can make custom shoes for patients with significant foot deformity. Some deformities, such as prominent bunions, can be accommodated by stretching the shoe uppers with a specially designed tool. Finally, some individuals with weakness or instability at the joints of the foot or ankle may need wedges or flares built into the shoe or braces that can improve stability and/or transfer some load from the foot to the leg. Shoe size (length and width) must be determined by measurement, because a neuropathic patient can never be depended on to give an accurate impression of how the shoes fit.

Table 4.1 General Guide to Footwear Prescription Based on Risk Status

Deformity, prior plantar ulcer, callus, high plantar pressure	Activity		
	Low	Moderate	High
None	Sports shoe as is, or depth shoe with a soft insole	Sports or depth shoe with a thick insole	Sports or depth shoe with a thick insole; consider rocker bottom
Moderate	Sports or depth shoe with a thick insole	Sports or depth shoe with a thick insole; consider rocker bottom	Sports or depth shoe with a thick insole, rocker bottom; consider custom shoe with thicker insole, consider reliefs
Severe	Customized upper or custom shoe, thick insole	Customized upper or custom shoe, thick insole with reliefs, rocker bottom	Customized upper or custom shoe, thick insole with complex reliefs, rocker bottom

Choice of Insoles

Insoles for patients with loss of sensation should accommodate rather than "correct." Functional orthotics, the in-shoe devices that are widely used to correct foot alignment (in sports medicine, for example) tend to increase loading and are therefore typically not appropriate for neuropathic patients. The stock insoles delivered with most therapeutic shoes contain fillers and usually need to be replaced before the patient can wear the shoe. Flat insoles can deliver significant off-loading benefit as thickness increases, and patients with high-risk feet should use insoles of up to 3/8″ if there is room in the shoe. Insoles made with materials such as PPT or Spenco do not degrade markedly with use, unlike some common insole materials that rapidly "bottom out" and should no longer be used (19). Higher quality insoles in depth shoes can effectively reduce plantar pressure in patients without major foot deformity.

Custom insoles incorporating the load-relief strategies mentioned above are made by a pedorthist from an impression of the patient's foot shape. All insoles must precisely match the contour of the shoe in which they will be placed. Patients should be given several pairs of insoles when the shoes are dispensed so that they can use them in rotation. Thick socks (similar to sport socks) are also effective in reducing pressure (20), but they must be used only when there is enough room in the shoes.

The Footwear Prescription

The following steps provide a useful approach to the therapeutic footwear prescription:

1. Determine intended use of the shoe—home, work, waterproof, all-weather outsole, etc.
2. Select the level of plantar protection required—thickness of insole, reliefs and supports, rocker bottom
3. Decide the volume of shoe needed to accommodate dorsal deformity and the insole selected—sports shoe, depth shoe, stretches and reliefs of the upper, custom-molded upper

4. Address stability issues—outsole flares, wedges, bracing, aids to walking

Medicare Guidelines

At the time of writing (September 2004), Medicare reimburses the provider $100.80 for a pair of depth shoes, $302.40 for custom shoes, and $51.20 for a pair of insoles. For the patient to be eligible for the Medicare Diabetic Therapeutic Footwear benefit, the treating physician must provide a written statement certifying that at least one of the following conditions exists:

- history of partial or complete amputation of the foot
- history of previous foot ulceration
- history of preulcerative calluses
- peripheral neuropathy with evidence of callus formation
- foot deformity
- poor circulation

This statement must be kept on file by the supplier, along with a prescription ordering the diabetic footwear, insoles, and other devices. Coverage in one calendar year is provided for one pair of custom-molded footwear plus two pairs of insoles, or one pair of extra-depth footwear and three pairs of insoles. Shoe modifications (such as wedges, flares, roller/rocker, metatarsal bars) may be substituted for a pair of insoles. The footwear must meet the Medicare definitions of depth or custom-molded shoes.

Other Footwear Issues

The very best prescription footwear is not effective if patients do not use it. Clinicians must educate their patients and provide attractive, socially acceptable shoes that protect against foot injury. Patients must understand that wearing the prescribed shoes falls into the same category as taking medication—something that is essential for preserving their health. The syndrome of the "holiday ulcer" is commonplace: many ulcers develop at weddings, funerals, religious events, or on vacation because the patient selects inappropriate footwear "just this once" and usually engages in increased activity. Compliance with wearing appropriate shoes and avoiding barefoot walking must be stressed at every office visit. Conversely, the clinician should explain to low-risk patients why they do not need specialized footwear.

At present, footwear prescription is often a trial-and-error process in which success is not assured. Patients should use a new prescription for short periods during the day, increasing the duration only when frequent inspection shows that no new injury is being caused. In the future, shoes and insoles designed according to functional measurements made directly from the patient's gait should increase the probability of successful prevention and provide reproducible and validated interventions.

Note

Details of Medicare coverage of therapeutic footwear for people with diabetes can be found at http://www.ndep.nih.gov/resources/feet/medicare.htm. Information on the Pedorthic Footwear Association can be found at http://www.pedorthics.org.

References

1. Reiber GE: The epidemiology of diabetic foot problems. *Diabet Med* 13 (Suppl. 1):S6–S11, 1996

2. Gey DC, Lesho EP, Manngold J: Management of peripheral arterial disease. *Am Fam Physician* 69:525–532, 2004; published erratum in *Am Fam Physician* 69: 1863, 2004

3. Price EW: Studies on plantar ulceration in leprosy. III. The natural history of plantar ulcers. *Lepr Rev* 30:180, 1959

4. Edmonds ME, Blundell MP, Morris ME, Thomas EM, Cotton LT, Watkins PJ: Improved survival of the diabetic foot: the role of a specialized foot clinic. *Q J Med* 60:763–771, 1986

5. Apelqvist J, Larsson J, Agardh CD: The influence of external precipitating factors and peripheral neuropathy on the development and outcome of diabetic foot ulcers. *J Diabet Complications* 4:21–25, 1990

6. Reiber GE: Who is at risk for limb loss and what to do about it? Clinical report. *J Rehabil Res Dev* 31:357–362, 1994

7. MacFarlane RM, Jeffcoate WJ: Factors contributing to the presentation of diabetic foot ulcers. *Diabet Med* 14:867–870, 1997

8. Uccioli L, Faglia E, Monticone G, Favales F, Durola L, Aldeghi A, Quarantiello A, Calia P, Menzinger G: Manufactured shoes in the prevention of diabetic foot ulcers. *Diabetes Care* 18:1376–1377, 1995

9. Chantelau E, Kushner T, Spraul M: How effective is cushioned therapeutic footwear in protecting diabetic feet? A clinical study. *Diabet Med* 7:355–359, 1990

10. Murray HJ, Young MJ, Hollis S, Boulton AJ: The association between callus formation, high pressures and neuropathy in diabetic foot ulceration. *Diabet Med* 13:979–982, 1996

11. Busch K, Chantelau E: Effectiveness of a new brand of stock "diabetic" shoes to protect against diabetic foot ulcer relapse: a prospective cohort study. *Diabet Med* 20:665–669, 2003

12. Viswanathan V, Madhavan S, Gnanasundaram S, Gopalakrishna G, Das BN, Rajasekar S, Ramachandran A: Effectiveness of different types of footwear insoles for the diabetic neuropathic foot: a follow-up study. *Diabetes Care* 27:474–477, 2004

13. Litzelman DK, Marriott DJ, Vinicor F: The role of footwear in the prevention of foot lesions in patients with NIDDM. *Diabetes Care* 20:156–162, 1997

14. Reiber GE, Smith DG, Wallace C, Sullivan K, Hayes S, Vath C, Maciejewski ML, Yu O, Heagerty PJ, LeMaster J: Effect of therapeutic footwear on foot reulceration in patients with diabetes. *JAMA* 287:2552–2558, 2002

15. Wooldridge J, Bergeron J, Thornton C: Preventing diabetic foot disease: lessons from the Medicare therapeutic shoe demonstration. *Am J Public Health* 86:935–938, 1996

16. Perry JE, Ulbrecht JS, Derr JA, Cavanagh PR: The use of running shoes to reduce plantar pressures in patients who have diabetes. *J Bone Joint Surg* 77A:1819–1828, 1995

17. Soulier SM: The use of running shoes in the prevention of plantar diabetic ulcers. *J Am Podiatr Med Assoc* 76:395–400, 1986

18. van Schie C, Ulbrecht JS, Becker MB, Cavanagh PR: Design criteria for rigid rocker shoes. *Foot Ankle Int* 21:833–844, 2000

19. Foto JG, Birke JA: Evaluation of multidensity orthotic materials used in footwear for patients with diabetes. *Foot Ankle Int* 19:836–841, 1998

20. Veves A, Masson EA, Fernando DJ, Boulton AJ: Use of experimental padded hosiery to reduce abnormal foot pressures in diabetic neuropathy. *Diabetes Care* 12:653–655, 1989

5

Ulcer Assessment and Classification

Nicolaas C. Schaper, MD

I N DIABETIC PATIENTS, the foot is the crossroad of several patho-
logical processes. Almost all components of the lower extremity are
involved: skin, subcutaneous tissue, muscles, bones, joints, blood vessels, and nerves (1). Because each of these components can contribute
to foot ulcers, a multidisciplinary approach is needed, and a standardized assessment is essential to guide further diagnostic work-up and
therapy. A diabetic foot ulcer is here defined as any "full-thickness"
lesion of the skin—that is, a wound penetrating through the dermis.
Lesions such as blisters or skin mycosis are not defined as ulcers (1).

Standardized Assessment

One of the pitfalls in assessing a foot ulcer is the limited value of history taking. If patients have loss of sensation, limited mobility, and
poor vision, they may not even be aware that they have a foot ulcer.
In addition, both patient and clinician can mistakenly be reassured
by the paucity of ulcer symptoms. However, the absence of symptoms generally does not rule out infection or critical limb ischemia,
and symptoms such as fever or pain suggest severe problems, neces-
sitating extensive evaluation.

Perfusion (Ischemia and Critical Limb Ischemia)

Claudication and ischemic rest pain are absent in many ischemic foot ulcers, probably due to sensory neuropathy, but if they are present, the risk of amputation is greatly enhanced and an aggressive vascular evaluation should be performed. In all patients, the proximal vessels, particularly the iliofemoral segment, should be auscultated for bruits. The pulses of the femoral, popliteal, dorsalis pedis, and posterior tibial artery should be palpated; if both foot arteries can be felt, severe ischemia is unlikely. However, palpation of foot pulses is not always reliable, and patients with palpable pulses can still have severe peripheral arterial disease (PAD) (2). Therefore, further noninvasive tests should be performed if the wound has no healing tendency in 3 weeks despite optimal therapy (1).

Additional signs of severe ischemia are multiple sites of skin necrosis, gangrene, and blanching of the feet when they are elevated, with a red-purple discoloration when the patient is standing or when the leg is in dependency. The feet can be red and warm despite severe ischemia, probably due to the relative high shunt blood flow, a consequence of autonomic neuropathy.

Noninvasive vascular evaluation is needed if ulcers do not heal, if one or two pulses are not palpable, or if other signs of ischemia are present (2–4). Measuring the systolic arterial pressure at the ankle with a handheld Doppler is a simple screening test, but ankle arteries can become less compressible due to media calcification, resulting in falsely elevated pressures. Systolic toe pressures probably predict wound healing more reliably. Transcutaneous oxygen pressure ($tcPO_2$) can give additional information on the probability of wound healing.

An ankle-brachial index of <0.9, a toe-brachial index of <0.6, or a $tcPO_2$ <60 mmHg suggests an ischemic or a neuroischemic ulcer. Critical limb ischemia is probably present when ankle pressure is <50 mmHg, a toe pressure is <30 mmHg, or a $tcPO_2$ is <20–30 mmHg. If clinical and/or noninvasive assessments suggest significant PAD, a vascular surgeon should be consulted and revascularization considered. Microvascular abnormalities do not play a major role in the pathogenesis of diabetic foot ulcers, and micro-angiopathy is no excuse for poorly healing wounds.

Depth, Size, and Location

The location of an ulcer can give clues to its cause and will help to determine if and how pressure relief should be applied. Neuropathic ulcers are usually located on areas with elevated pressure, such as the plantar side of the foot; ischemic or neuroischemic ulcers are more common on the tips of the toes or the lateral border. Because the ulcer is frequently covered by callus or necrotic tissue, the extent of tissue loss should be evaluated after initial debridement, but this should be performed judiciously when critical limb ischemia is suspected. Because of neuropathy, anesthesia is usually not necessary. In clinical practice, ulcers can be divided into two types: lesions confined to the skin (superficial) and those with tissue loss or infection deeper than the skin (deep) (1).

Infection

Infection of the diabetic foot is one of the major reasons for lower-extremity amputation. Unfortunately, no gold standard exists for diag-nosing an infection, and signs can be subtle, despite extensive tissue destruction. A superficial infection (not extending through the fascia) without systemic signs can be diagnosed based on local swelling, puru-lent discharge, erythema, foul smell, or local tenderness or pain. A swab of the surface of the ulcer is of little value for microbiological diagnosis because the ulcer is usually colonized by various microorganisms (1). Preferably, pus or a curettement of the ulcer base is obtained after debridement. Systemic signs—such as elevated white blood cell count, erythrocyte sedimentation rate, or body temperature—are frequently absent in deep infections (extending through the skin). If systemic signs are present, there could be a foot abscess.

Osteomyelitis can also pose diagnostic problems. With an infected ulcer, if bone is probed before debridement, the risk of osteomyelitis is increased. An X-ray should be considered for any infected ulcer, but it may take several weeks before radiological changes appear, and a normal X-ray does not exclude osteomyelitis. A repeat X-ray after 2–4 weeks can be helpful, but X-rays are not very specific. Bone scans are more sensitive, but again, specificity is relatively low. MRIs are currently considered the most accurate imaging technique (1,4). A more-definitive diagnosis can be obtained with a bone biopsy (4).

Sensation, Biomechanical Evaluation, and Immediate Cause

Polyneuropathy is a major factor in foot ulceration, resulting in loss of protective sensation, muscle paralysis with subsequent deformities, abnormal walking patterns, and abnormal loading of the foot. The Semmes-Weinstein monofilament is a simple tool to assess loss of sensation. This inexpensive instrument consists of a fiber that buckles at a standardized pressure force, such as 10 g; usually a 10-g monofilament is applied. The monofilament should be placed perpendicular to the surface of the skin, as described in Chapter 2. Vibration perception, determined with a 128-Hz tuning fork at the hallux, is an additional simple test (1).

Callus and foot deformities—such as hallux valgus, prominent metatarsal heads, or clawing of the toes—are easily recognized during inspection of the feet, which should be performed with the patient both supine and standing. Abnormalities near an ulcer suggest increased biomechanical stress as a direct cause. Mobility in the first toe (hallux rigidus) and in the ankle joint should be estimated in plantar ulcerations, but these measurements are difficult to standardize. Finally, both of the shoes and socks should be examined. The fit of the footwear is especially important to evaluate, as most ulcers are caused by poorly fitting shoes and insoles.

Classification

Various systems have been proposed to classify diabetic foot ulcers, such as the Meggitt-Wagner system, the University of Texas (UT) system and the S(AD) SAD system (see Table 5.1). Unfortunately,

Table 5.1 Three Classification Schemes for Foot Ulcers

Meggitt-Wagner System

Grade

0. Pre-ulcerative/high-risk foot
1. Superficial ulcer
2. Deep to tendon, bone, or joint
3. Deep with abscess/osteomyelitis
4. Forefoot gangrene
5. Whole foot gangrene

UT System

Grade

1. Pre- or postulcerative lesion	Stage A–D
2. Superficial	Stage A–D
3. Penetrates to tendon or capsule	Stage A–D
4. Penetrates to bone	Stage A–D

Stages: A = no infection or ischemia; B = infection; C = ischemia; D = infection and ischemia

PEDIS System

Perfusion	Normal signs / Moderate ischemia / Critical limb ischemia
Extent	Area in cm^2
Depth	Superficial / Subcutaneous, no bone / Deep, extends to bone
Infection	No infection / Superficial and localized / Extensive or deep / Systemic involvement
Sensation	Normal / Abnormal

none has gained universal acceptance (5–7). The UT system is a validated extension of the well-known Wagner system and includes such vital items as depth and the presence of ischemia or infection; it also gives information about the risk of amputation from an individual ulcer (6). One of the attractions of this system is that it underlines the poor prognosis of the combination of ischemia and infection. The

PEDIS system was recently developed by an international consensus group for research purposes; this system, which was used in this chapter, gives criteria for several abnormalities (4).

Summary

Describing a wound in the foot of diabetic patient as a "diabetic foot ulcer" is too vague. It is not a diagnosis and does not give any information on prognosis. Instead, all foot ulcers in diabetic patients should be evaluated following a rigid and standard protocol. Ulcers can be described as

- neuropathic, neuroischemic, or ischemic, with or without critical limb ischemia
- superficial or deep
- infected or not infected

In addition, the following aspects should be summarized:

- site of the ulcer (e.g., under head of MTP1 or on dorsal side of toe)
- extent (preferably in cm^2)
- immediate cause (e.g., increased biomechanical stress because of prominent MTP1 or an acute trauma from walking barefoot)

These data will provide the basis for the initial diagnosis and are the cornerstones for formulating a management plan.

References

1. International Working Group on the Diabetic Foot: *International Consensus on the Diabetic Foot.* Amsterdam, Netherlands, International Diabetes Federation, 1999

2. TransAtlantic Inter-Society Consensus (TASC): Management of peripheral arterial disease (PAD). *Eur J Vasc Endovasc Surg* 19 (Suppl. A):Si–Sxxviii, S1–S250, 2000

3. Schaper NC, Kitslaar PJEM: Peripheral vascular disease in diabetes. In *International Textbook of Diabetes Mellitus.* 3rd ed. De Fronzo R, Ferrannini E, Keen H, Zimmet P, Eds. New York, John Wiley and Sons, 2004

4. Schaper NC: Diabetic foot ulcer classification system for research purposes: a progress report on criteria for including patients in research studies. *Diabetes Metab Res Rev* 20 (Suppl. 1):S90–S95, 2004

5. Wagner FW: The dysvascular foot: a system for diagnosis and treatment. *Foot Ankle* 2:64–122, 1981

6. Armstrong DG, Lavery LA, Harkless LB: Validation of a diabetic wound classification system: the contribution of depth, infection, and ischemia to risk of amputation. *Diabetes Care* 21:855–859, 1998

7. Macfarlane RM, Jeffcoate WJ: Classification of diabetic foot ulcers: the S(AD) SAD system. *The Diabetic Foot* 2:123–131, 1999

6

Off-Loading the Diabetic Foot Wound

David G. Armstrong, DPM, PhD, MSc
Stephanie Wu, DPM

N EUROPATHIC DIABETIC FOOT WOUNDS are caused by a combination of focal pressure and repetitive stress at a given site (1). Pressure relief, via debridement and off-loading, is therefore fundamental in treating neuropathic diabetic foot wounds. Because the amount of pressure exerted is inversely proportional to the area of the body on which it rests, strategies for relieving pressure generally involve spreading a finite amount of force across the largest possible area. Some of the most common off-loading modalities are described here.

The Edge Effect

Maximum soft tissue damage often occurs at the edge, not the center, of pressure sites (1). This tissue damage around a bony prominence that occurs secondary to repetitive vertical stress and shear is known as the edge effect (2). The edge effect leads to increased inflammation, hyperemia, and stimulation of fibroblasts, which causes new skin and callus to be formed. The increased pressure provokes further inflammation, thus continuing a vicious cycle.

Crutches, Walkers, and Wheelchairs

Although crutches and walkers are excellent devices to off-load a foot completely, they are less effective among patients with diabetes. Most diabetic patients with foot ulcerations do not have the upper body strength, the endurance, or the will to use them. Patients often do not perceive any functional limitations in their ulcerated limb, so they tend to be noncompliant. Plus, some of the devices can increase pressure on the unaffected side and place the contralateral limb at risk for ulceration (1). Although wheelchairs serve as a good alternative to either crutches or walkers, most patients' homes are not designed for wheelchair access, thus reducing their usefulness in the place where most daily activity occurs.

Therapeutic Footwear (Depth Inlay Shoes)

Therapeutic shoes and insoles are probably better at preventing ulcers than at healing active ones. Gait studies suggest that therapeutic shoes allow up to 900% more pressure in areas of the forefoot compared with total contact casts and some removable cast walkers (3,4).

Half Shoes

Half shoes (Fig. 6.1) were originally designed to decrease pressure on the forefoot postoperatively (5) and have become quite popular for treatment of diabetic foot wounds, because they are inexpensive and easy to apply. Compared with patients treated with a regimen of routine wound care and use of crutches, patients placed in half shoes healed 59% faster and developed fewer serious infections. Half shoes, however, are much less effective at reducing pressure than total contact casts and certain removable cast walkers.

Healing Sandals

Theoretically, adding a rigid rocker to the sole of a specially designed sandal limits plantar progression of the metatarsal heads during

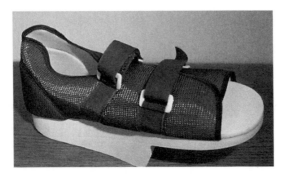

Figure 6.1 The half shoe.

propulsion in gait and provides greater distribution of pressure on the metatarsal head and a shorter pressure-time integral. This device is lightweight, stable, and reusable, but it takes time and experience to produce and modify it. In addition, it doesn't off-load as well as other modalities (such as removable cast walkers) that are easier to produce or procure (6).

MABAL Shoe

Recently developed, the MABAL shoe is a cross between a healing sandal and a Scotchcast boot. The device is removable but maintains more contact with the foot than a standard healing sandal does. In a study by Hissink et al. (7), healing time with this device was similar to total contact casting. However, the MABAL shoe is like the contact cast and healing sandal in that special expertise is needed to make and apply it.

Casts

Scotchcast Boot

The Scotchcast boot is a well-padded, ankle-high cast aimed at reducing plantar pressure while maintaining patient mobility and protecting the rest of the foot. The boot can be made removable by cutting away the cast over the dorsum of the foot and making a closure of padding and tape with Velcro straps. Windows are cut over the ulcers as needed, and a removable heel cap of fiberglass is added for large heel ulcers. The boot is worn with a cast sandal to increase the patient's mobility while protecting the ulcer from pressure during ambulation. The Scotchcast boot is light, has high integral strength, and is used as an alternative to plaster of Paris (8). Removable Scotchcast boots allow regular inspection and redressing of the wound, but if patient compliance is an issue, then nonremovable ones should be applied.

Although Scotchcast boots have been used successfully for more than a decade in several British clinics, mostly for treating neuropathic or neuroischemic ulcers, no studies comparing healing rates of this type of cast with the more standard casts, such as the total contact cast, have been done. Preliminary data of healing rates ranging from 61% to 88%, with a mean healing time between 10 and 13 weeks, have been reported (8,9).

Total Contact Casts

Most diabetic foot specialists consider total contact casts (Fig. 6.2) the gold standard of the off-loading modalities (10). Treatment of neuropathic foot wounds via plaster casting was first described by Milroy Paul and later popularized in the United States by Dr. Paul Brand at the Hansen's Disease Center in Carville, Louisiana (11). The technique is known as total contact casting because it employs

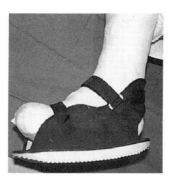

Figure 6.2 The total contact cast.

a well-molded, minimally padded cast that maintains contact with the entire plantar aspect of the foot and the lower leg. Total contact casting permits walking by uniformly distributing pressure over the entire plantar surface of the foot (11–18). It effectively treats most noninfected, nonischemic plantar diabetic foot wounds, with healing rates ranging from 72% to 100% over a course of 5–7 weeks (15–20).

In addition to off-loading, total contact casts may help reduce or control edema, which can impede healing, and can help protect the foot from infection (21). But perhaps the best thing about the total contact cast is that it ensures patient compliance, because it is not easily removable.

Unfortunately, most centers do not have a physician or cast technician with adequate training or experience to safely apply a total contact cast. Because improper cast application can cause skin irritation and in some cases even frank ulceration, this is its single biggest negative feature. These casts also do not allow daily wound assessment and care, so they are generally contraindicated in wounds with soft tissue infections or osteomyelitis. In addition, patients in total contact casts may have difficulty bathing without getting the cast wet and trouble sleeping comfortably. Moreover, certain designs may exacerbate postural instability (22).

Removable Cast Walkers

Removable cast walkers (Fig. 6.3) such as the Aircast or the DH Pressure Relief Walker are just as effective as total contact casts in reducing pressure. Removable cast walkers permit daily inspection and wound care and can therefore be used for both infected wounds and superficial ulcers. However, being removable eliminates the element of forced compliance, which is the best thing about the total contact casts. Patients may remove the cast for dressing changes, sleeping, and showers, but they can also choose to use the walker only when they leave the house or walk excessively. Because of this, removable cast walkers lag significantly behind the total contact cast in prevalence and rate of healing.

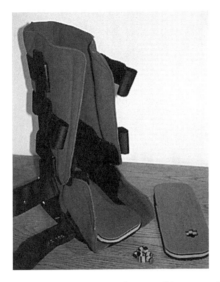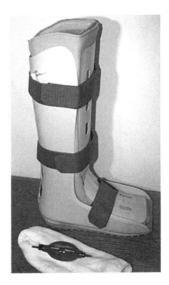

Figure 6.3 Two types of removable cast walkers.

Instant Total Contact Cast

Armstrong and others have developed a simple, rapid technique to convert a removable cast walker into a device that is less easily removed by simply wrapping the cast walker with cohesive bandage or plaster of Paris (Fig. 6.4). This modification takes less time and costs less than total contact casts, which need to be reapplied. It requires very little training to apply and is reusable. Recent data suggest that the instant total contact cast may heal wounds faster than a standard removable cast walker and at a similar rate to traditional total contact casts (23,24).

Summary

Pressure relief via off-loading is essential to healing foot ulcers. Crutches, walkers, and wheelchairs provide complete off-loading, but noncompliance and inaccessibility in the home are factors that detract from them. Therapeutic footwear reduces pressure, but some

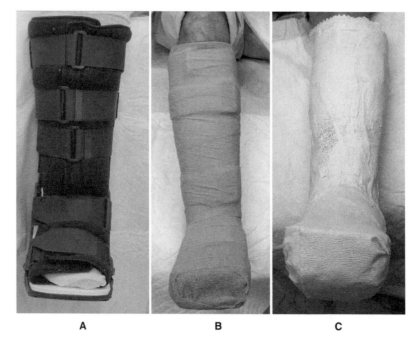

Figure 6.4 The instant total contact cast. A removable cast walker (A) can easily be converted into an instant total cast by wrapping it with a cohesive bandage (B) or plaster of Paris (C).

types require an expert to apply them. Casts like the Scotchcast boot, total contact, removable cast walker, or instant total contact all effectively off-load pressure. Some, such as the total contact cast and instant total contact cast, ensure patient compliance because they can't be removed, thus increasing healing rates.

References

1. Brand PW: The diabetic foot. In *Diabetes Mellitus, Theory and Practice.* 3rd ed. Ellenberg M, Rifkin H, Eds. New York, Medical Examination Publishing, 1983, p. 803–828

2. Armstrong DG, Athanasiou KA: The edge effect: how and why wounds grow in size and depth. *Clin Podiatr Med Surg* 15:105–108, 1998

3. Armstrong DG, Liswood PL, Todd WF: The contralateral limb during total contact casting: a dynamic pressure and thermometric analysis. *J Am Podiatr Med Assoc* 85:733–737, 1995

4. Lavery LA, Vela SA, Lavery DC, Quebedeaux TL: Reducing dynamic foot pressures in high-risk diabetic subjects with foot ulcerations. A comparison of treatments. *Diabetes Care* 19:818–821, 1996

5. Chantelau E, Breuer U, Leisch AC, Tanudjada T, Reuter M: Outpatient treatment of unilateral diabetic foot ulcers with "half shoes." *Diabet Med* 10:267–270, 1993

6. Giacalone VF, Armstrong DG, Ashry HR, Lavery DC, Harkless LB, Lavery LA: A quantitative assessment of healing sandals and postoperative shoes in off-loading the neuropathic diabetic foot. *J Foot Ankle Surg* 36:28–30, 1997

7. Hissink RJ, Manning HA, van Baal JG: The MABAL shoe, an alternative method in contact casting for the treatment of neuropathic diabetic foot ulcers. *Foot Ankle Int* 21:320–323, 2000

8. Burden AC, Jones GR, Jones R, Blandford RL: Use of the "Scotchcast boot" in treating diabetic foot ulcers. *Br Med J (Clin Res Ed)* 286:1555–1557, 1983

9. Knowles A, Boulton AJM: Use of the Scotchcast boot to heal diabetic foot ulcers. *Proceedings of the 5th European Conference of Advanced Wound Care*, London, 1996

10. American Diabetes Association: Consensus Development Conference on Diabetic Foot Wound Care. *Diabetes Care* 22:1354–1360, 1999

11. Coleman W, Brand PW, Birke JA: The total contact cast, a therapy for plantar ulceration on insensitive feet. *J Am Podiatry Assoc* 74:548–552, 1984

12. Boulton AJ, Bowker JH, Gadia M, Lemerman R, Caswell K, Skyler JS, Sosenko JM: Use of plaster casts in the management of diabetic neuropathic foot ulcers. *Diabetes Care* 9:149–152, 1986

13. Kominsky SJ: The ambulatory total contact cast. In *The High Risk Foot in Diabetes Mellitus.* 1st ed. Frykberg RG, Ed. New York, Churchill Livingstone, 1991, p. 449–455

14. Lavery LA, Armstrong DG, Walker SC: Healing rates of diabetic foot ulcers associated with midfoot fracture due to Charcot's arthropathy. *Diabet Med* 14:46–49, 1997

15. Armstrong DG, Lavery LA, Bushman TR: Peak foot pressures influence the healing time of diabetic foot ulcers treated with total contact casts. *J Rehabil Res Dev* 35:1–5, 1998

16. Walker SC, Helm PA, Pulliam G: Chronic diabetic neuropathic foot ulcerations and total contact casting: healing effectiveness and outcome probability (Abstract). *Arch Phys Med Rehabil* 66:574, 1985

17. Walker SC, Helm PA, Pulliam G: Total contact casting and chronic diabetic neuropathic foot ulcerations: healing rates by wound location. *Arch Phys Med Rehabil* 68:217–221, 1987

18. Sinacore DR, Mueller MJ, Diamond JE: Diabetic plantar ulcers treated by total contact casting. *Phys Ther* 67:1543–1547, 1987

19. Myerson M, Papa J, Eaton K, Wilson K: The total contact cast for management of neuropathic plantar ulceration of the foot. *J Bone Joint Surg* 74A:261–269, 1992

20. Helm PA, Walker SC, Pulliam G: Total contact casting in diabetic patients with neuropathic foot ulcerations. *Arch Phys Med Rehabil* 65:691–693, 1984

21. Mueller MJ, Diamond JE, Sinacore DR, Delitto A, Blair VP, Drury DA, Rose SJ: Total contact casting in treatment of diabetic plantar ulcers. Controlled clinical trial (see comments). *Diabetes Care* 12:384–388, 1989

22. Lavery LA, Fleishli JG, Laughlin TJ, Vela SA, Lavery DC, Armstrong DG: Is postural instability exacerbated by off-loading devices in high risk diabetics with foot ulcers? *Ostomy Wound Manage* 44:26–32, 34, 1998

23. Katz IA, Harlan A, Miranda-Palma B, Prieto-Sanchez L, Armstrong DG, Bowker JH, Mizel MS, Boulton AJM: A randomized trial of two irremovable off-loading devices in the management of plantar neuropathic diabetic foot ulcers. *Diabetes Care.* In press

24. Armstrong DG, Lavery LA, Wu SC, Boulton AJM: Evaluation of removable and irremovable cast walkers in the healing of diabetic foot wounds: a randomized controlled trial. *Diabetes Care.* In press

7

Debridement of the Diabetic Foot

Christopher Attinger, MD

NECROTIC TISSUE, FOREIGN MATERIAL, AND BACTERIA in a wound impede the body's attempt to heal by producing or stimulating the production of metalloproteases such as collagenases and elastases. These then overwhelm the building blocks—chemotactants, growth factors, mitogens—needed for normal wound healing. This hostile environment enables bacteria to proliferate. The bacteria further inhibit healing by producing their own destructive enzymes, by producing a biofilm for protection, and by consuming the local resources necessary for healing (oxygen, nutrition, and building blocks).

Removing necrotic tissue, foreign material, and bacteria from an acute or chronic wound, known as debridement, is a critical step in allowing the wound to go through the normal phases of healing in a timely fashion. A recent wound that has yet to progress through the normal healing stages is acute; debriding an acute wound removes ischemic tissue and foreign material that would inhibit it from healing. A chronic wound is arrested in one of the healing stages (usually the inflammatory stage) and cannot progress further. Debriding the chronic wound to normal tissue converts it into an acute wound that can progress through the normal phases of healing.

Debridement is critical to the wound healing process. However, concerns about possible reconstruction problems all too often prevent the debrider from removing all the nonviable tissue. The extent of debridement should be determined by getting to the boundary of normal tissue and not by concerns of how to subsequently rebuild the foot. After adequate debridement, foot reconstruction should be guided by the growth of healthy new granulation tissue, by how much normal tissue is left behind, and by the biomechanical stability of the remaining structure.

Aggressive debridement is also required when applying wound healing adjuncts such as growth factors or live skin substitutes. Unless the adjuncts are placed on a clean, well-debrided, and adequately vascularized wound bed, growth factors are quickly inactivated by proteases, and cultured skin products are quickly digested.

Timing

When dealing with gangrene in the ischemic limb, the timing between debridement and revascularization is critical. When initially faced with wet gangrene, the wound should be debrided immediately, and the leg should be revascularized as soon as possible thereafter. If there is dry gangrene and no cellulitis, the limb should be revascularized first. It takes 4–10 days after revascularization to optimize blood flow to the foot. To avoid debriding potentially viable tissue during this time, debridement should be delayed until the wound has developed maximal blood flow from the new bypass. However, if the dry gangrene converts to wet gangrene before full tissue revascularization has occurred, the gangrene should be immediately debrided.

Debride well-vascularized wounds immediately if wet gangrene is present. If there is evidence of new tissue growth underneath dry gangrene, observe the gangrene until it falls off or converts to wet gangrene and needs to be debrided. If there is no evidence of healing underneath the dry gangrene, it should be debrided.

Surgical Debridement

When debriding, use atraumatic surgical techniques to avoid damaging the healthy tissue left behind. Such tissue will be the future source of growth factors, nutrients, and the building blocks required for subsequent healing, and it should be protected. To leave a maximal amount of viable tissue behind, avoid traumatizing techniques such as crushing the skin edges with forceps or clamps, burning tissue with electrocautery, or tying off large clumps of tissue with sutures.

The principal debriding technique consists of removing the grossly contaminated or ischemic tissue en masse. Use any appropriate surgical tool, including a surgical blade, mayo scissors, curettes, or rongeurs. However, as you get close to the viable tissue, slice thin layer of tissue after thin layer of tissue until only normal tissue remains. This technique minimizes the amount of viable tissue sacrificed while ensuring that the tissue left behind will be healthy. Recently available is a hydrosurgical debrider that uses a water jet with up to 15,000 psi to debride tissue. The Venturi effect caused by this high pressure water jet sucks tissue into the stream of water, thus separating it from underlying tissue. The debrider works rapidly to take thin slice after thin slice of tissue with minimal surrounding tissue trauma.

The basic tools of debridement used in an office include pickups, knife, scissors, and a curette. Surgical tools, not disposable suture removal kits, are recommended because the latter are usually dull, and they crush and damage the normal tissue left behind. Grasp the tissue to be removed with the pickup and use a #10 or #20 blade to slice off tissue, thin layer by thin layer (Fig. 7.1), until you reach healthy tissue. Change surgical blades frequently, as they dull quickly. Curettes with sharp edges are very helpful for removing the proteinaceous coagulum that accumulates on top of both fresh and chronic granulation tissue (Fig. 7.2, A and B). Rongeurs are useful for removing hard-to-reach soft tissue and for debriding bone. An air-driven or electrical sagittal saw can serially saw off bone until you

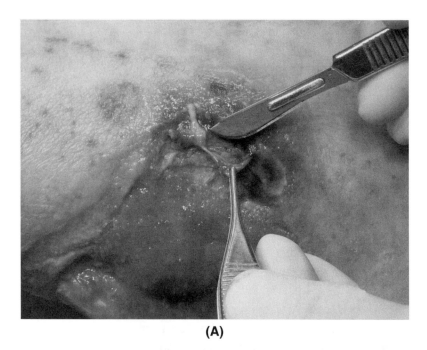

(A)

(B)

Figure 7.1 Remove thin slices of necrotic tissue, one at a time (A). The appearance of clotted veins in the tissue (B) signifies that further debridement (C) is needed. Continue debriding until only normal tissue is left behind (D). (continued)

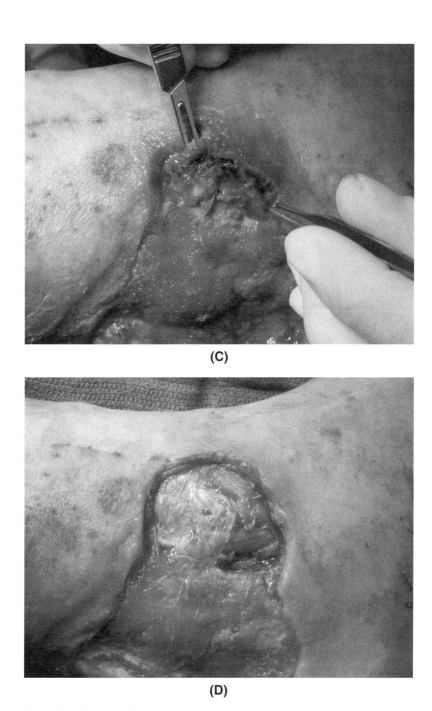

(C)

(D)

Figure 7.1 (*Continued*)

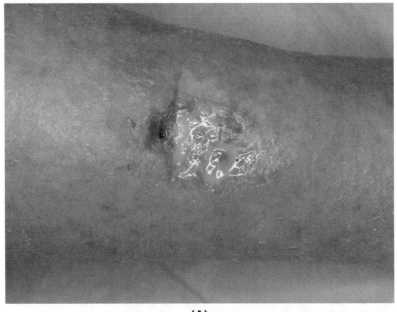

(A)

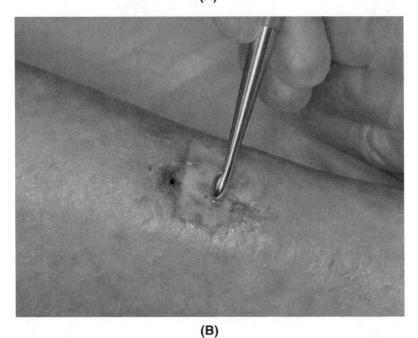

(B)

Figure 7.2 The thick coagulum (A) that covers chronic and acute wounds should be curetted off (B, C) because it contains metalloproteases and bacterial biofilm that inhibit healing. After the wound is adequately curetted, only healthy granulating tissue should remain (D).

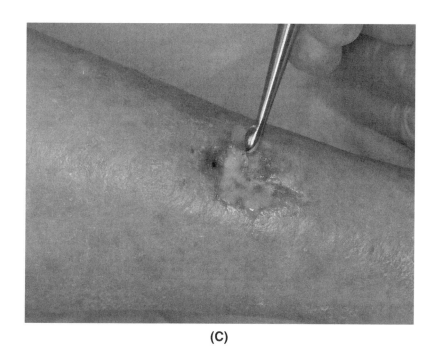

(C)

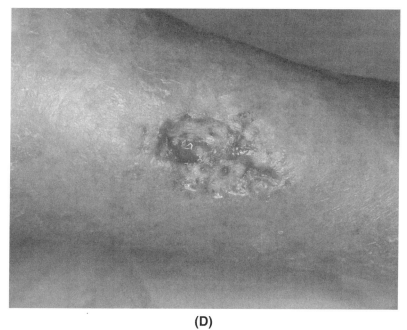

(D)

Figure 7.2 (*Continued*)

reach normal cortex and marrow. Cutting burrs and rasps permit fine debridement of bone surface until you see the telltale punctate bleeding at the freshened bone surface.

Debriding Skin

Remove nonviable skin as soon as possible. If the border between live and dead tissue is clearly demarcated, excise the skin along that border. If the border is not obvious, start at the center and remove concentric circles of skin until you reach bleeding tissue. When excising skin, look for bleeding at the normal skin edge. Clotted venules at the skin edge indicate that the local microcirculation has been completely interrupted and that further excision is necessary. Only when there is normal arterial and venous bleeding at the edge of the wound can you be satisfied that the cutaneous debridement has been adequate.

Debriding Subcutaneous Tissue

Subcutaneous tissue consists of fat, vessels, and nerves. Because of the decreased concentration of blood vessels in the subcutaneous fat, bleeding at the tissue's edge is not always a reliable indicator. Healthy fat has a shiny yellow color and is soft and resilient. Dead fat has a gray pallor to it, is hard, and is not pliable. Debride fat until you reach soft, yellow, normal-looking fat. After debridement, fat must be kept in a moist environment to prevent desiccation.

To minimize damage to the surrounding tissue, coagulate the small blood vessels using bipolar cautery. Ligate the vessels if they are larger than 2–3 mm. Ligaclips are the least-reactive foreign body material for this. If you are using a suture, a small-diameter monofilament suture will minimize the risk of further infection.

Debriding Fascia, Tendon, and Muscle

Healthy fascia has a hard, white, glistening appearance. When dead, it looks dull, soft, and stringy and is in the process of liquefying.

Debride all necrotic fascia until you reach solid, normal-looking bleeding fascia. The viable fascia must be kept moist during the post-debridement period to avoid desiccation.

Infected necrotic tendon looks dull, soft, and partially liquefied. To ensure that any hidden necrotic tendon is also removed, make a proximal and distal incision along the path of the exposed tendon. When the extensor tendons on the dorsum of the foot become exposed, it is hard to preserve them unless they are quickly covered with healthy tissue. If the tendons remain in place while the wound progresses and is ready to be closed, they usually become infected and will impede further healing until they are removed. With the larger Achilles or anterior tibial tendon, debride only the portion that is necrotic or infected. Leave the hard, shiny tendon underneath intact. The remaining tendon must be kept moist and clean, as it will granulate in. The tendon can then be skin grafted. Granulation formulation can be accelerated with the VAC (first cover the tendon with a Vaseline mesh gauze), a dermal template, cultured skin substitutes, or the combined use of topical growth factor and hyperbaric oxygen.

Examine the underlying muscle. Healthy muscle has a bright red, shiny, and resilient appearance, and it contracts when grasped with forceps or touched with cautery. In neuropathic patients, the muscle may have a pale, possibly yellowish, color and may appear nonviable. It will have some tone, however, and it bleeds when cut. Frankly dead muscle will be swollen, dull, and grainy when palpated, and it falls apart when pinched. If the muscle's viability is questionable, err on the side of caution and remove only what is not bleeding and appears dead. Subsequently, serially debride the wound until only viable muscle remains.

Debriding Bone

The key to debriding bone is to remove only what is dead and infected and leave hard bleeding bone behind. Be careful not to shatter proximal viable bone. In this regard, power tools are safer to use than rongeurs or chisels. The best way to debride the osteomyelitic smaller long bones (phalanx, metacarpals, or metatarsals) is to cut slices of bone serially until you reach healthy bone. In the larger bones, use a cutting burr to remove thin layer by thin layer of bone until you see punctate bleeding (paprika sign). Copiously irrigate to ensure that the heat generated by the burr does not damage the healthy bone. When debriding, continue until you reach marrow that is bleeding and appears normal.

Obtain cultures of normal bone near the area of debridement as well as of the debrided osteomyelitic bone. Once you remove the infected bone and only bleeding, healthy bone remains, the wound is ready to close, assuming that the surrounding soft tissue is also healthy. When only healthy, noninfected bone is left behind, just 1 week of appropriate antibiotics is necessary after wound closure. Only when you suspect that the bone left behind (e.g., calcaneus or tibia) may still harbor osteomyelitis is a longer course of antibiotics required.

Nonsurgical Modes of Debridement

Wet-to-dry dressing, where the moist gauze is allowed to dry on the wound and then ripped off, is the standard debriding dressing. Although this effectively removes dead tissue, it can lead to wound desiccation, can harm the viable tissue left behind, and is very painful in the sensate patient. Topical enzymatic debriding agents are effective, but they work slowly and can be painful. (If painful, they can be cut with a wound gel.)

The most effective debriding agent of all is to apply maggots to the wound. Thirty maggots consume 1 g tissue/day, consuming only necrotic tissue and bacteria and leaving all viable tissue intact. Maggots are painless and are very effective locally against antibiotic-resistant organisms. However, to use them, you need cooperation from both the patient and hospital staff.

Postdebridement

For extensive infection, with or without necrosis, repeat debridement every 12–48 hours until the wound is free of infection. This aggressive approach is often the only chance to save the diffusely infected limb. When the blood supply is adequate, progressive tissue necrosis after debridement usually represents lingering uncontrolled infection and indicates that further debridement is needed. Supplemental hyperbaric oxygen may be needed for necrotizing fasciitis.

Summary

Debridement is the key to enabling acute or chronic wounds to go through the normal healing process. An aggressive approach is sometimes needed to create a healing environment and to avoid amputation. Never condemn a limb to amputation too quickly, even if the amount of infection and necrosis requires extensive debridement. The debridement process may leave the foot and leg with what appears to be a formidable reconstructive challenge. However, with modern reconstructive techniques (i.e., plastic surgery and the Ilizarov frame), a functional limb can usually be fashioned. In addition, short foot amputations, such as Lisfranc or Chopart amputations, are viable options with the appropriate footwear to accommodate them.

Bibliography

Armstrong DG, Lavery LA, Nixon BP, Boulton AJ: It's not what you put on, but what you take off: techniques for debriding and off-loading the diabetic foot wound. *Clin Infect Dis* 39 (Suppl. 2):S92–S99, 2004

Attinger CE, Bulan E, Blume PA: Surgical debridement: the key to successful wound healing and reconstruction. *Clin Podiatr Med Surg* 17:599–630, 2000

8

Adjunctive Wound Therapies

Robert Kirsner, MD, PhD
Paul E. Banwell, BSc (Hon), MB, BS, FRCS

A DJUNCTIVE THERAPIES—the use of dressings and other wound healing therapies—form an important component of the holistic management of the diabetic foot. They augment and optimize the outcome of complex diabetic foot problems, and clinicians should be conversant with the range of modalities and therapies available. Along with debridement and off-loading, adjunctive therapies form an important triad of treatment. Close liaison with all members of the multidisciplinary team is required throughout the process.

Adjunctive therapies can be classified as either passive or active. Passive therapies include dressings that have various functions but do not actively modulate the wound healing environment. By contrast, active therapies include treatments that pharmacologically or physically modulate the wound environment.

Passive Therapies

Dressings

In combination with mechanical debridement, dressings can assist in the cleansing and sloughing of chronic wounds. Their primary purpose is to maintain a moist wound environment, which is conducive to healing via promotion of epithelialization. In addition, they protect the wound from external infection and trauma and absorb exudate to prevent maceration (when appropriate)—without adhering to the wound. (Table 8.1 provides a summary of indications and appropriate dressings.) Consider the following criteria when choosing dressings:

- Appearance of the wound: presence of necrosis, slough, granulation tissue, or epithelialization
- Exudate: viscosity and volume
- Appearance of the skin around the wound, e.g., is there maceration?
- Depth: cavity wound vs. superficial ulceration
- Odor
- Patient compliance
- Patient allergies and intolerance of products previously used
- Cost

Dressings may be divided into the following broad groups:

- *Low-adherent dressings* include Melolin, paraffin gauze-based products, and silicone-based products.
- *Semipermeable films* are permeable to gases and vapor but impermeable to liquids and bacteria. These dressings usually have an adhesive backing and provide a moist, ideal wound environment; they are usually not suitable for heavily exudative wounds.
- *Hydrogels* are composed of a starch polymer matrix; they swell to absorb moisture and exudates. They also promote autolysis of necrotic material and slough and hence are useful alternatives or adjuncts to sharp debridement.
- *Alginate dressings* are derived from seaweed. They contain calcium, which activates the clotting cascade when mixed with sodium within the wound. They are very absorbent, becoming gelatinous upon absorbing moisture.
- *Synthetic foams* are generally used in concave wounds and can conform to cavities, thus obliterating any potential dead space. They are suitable for heavily exudative wounds.

Table 8.1 Summary of Indications for Different Dressings

Appearance of the Wound	Therapeutic Alternatives
Presence of black, dry, necrotic tissue	Hydrogel Debridement
Presence of fibrin or moist necrotic tissue	Hydrocolloid Hydrogel, if little exudate Alginate, if heavily exuding
Cavity wound	Alginate ribbon Hydrocolloid gel Hydrocellular or foam pad
Heavily exuding wound	Alginate "New generation" hydrocolloid, hydrocellular, or foam
Granulating wound	Hydrocolloid Hydrocellular or foam Hydrogel Hydrofiber Alginate
Superficial wound or dermabrasion, superficial burn, donor graft site	Hydrocolloid Hydrocellular or foam Hydrogel Film Tulle and interface
Foul-smelling wound	Charcoal dressings
Infected wound	Alginate Charcoal dressings Silver-based dressings

Bioengineered Products

The development of skin substitutes heralded the first useful bioengineered products. They were originally designed for the massive skin loss associated with burns, but additional applications have evolved. Currently, two bioengineered skin products have been approved by the U.S. Food and Drug Administration (FDA) for treating diabetic foot ulcers. These cell therapies accelerate the closing of nonhealing, neuropathic ulcers. The first is Apligraf (or Graftskin; Organogenesis, Canton, MA), a bilayered skin equivalent, or human skin equivalent, which contains both allogeneic neonatal fibroblasts and keratinocytes. The second, a dermal equivalent that contains allogeneic neonatal fibroblasts seeded within a mesh scaffold, is called Dermagraft (Smith & Nephew, UK / Largo, FL).

Graftskin is made up of a cultured, living dermis and subsequently cultured epidermis whose cellular components are derived from neonatal foreskin. Applied weekly for up to 5 weeks, and followed for 12 weeks, the addition of Graftskin to a regimen of debridement and removable off-loading devices improved healing (56% vs. 38%, $P = 0.0042$) and reduced the incidence of osteomyelitis and lower-limb amputations (1).

A human fibroblast-derived dermis, Dermagraft is an allogeneic living dermal equivalent. In a trial that led to FDA approval, 30% of Dermagraft-treated patients, compared with 18.3% of the control patients, healed after 12 weeks. However, the low healing rates reported in the control group suggest that these patients either represented a particularly refractory group or, more likely, were noncompliant to off-loading (2).

Active Therapies

Topical Negative Pressure (Vacuum-Assisted Closure)

Topical negative pressure, or vacuum-assisted closure (VAC), has an important role in modulating the wound healing environment. A standard of care in treating many types of wounds, its use in diabetic wounds is encouraging. A physical, nonpharmacological method of actively stimulating granulation tissue formation, this therapy applies mechanical forces across the wound, thus improving local blood flow and reducing edema. Furthermore, it removes wound exudate and reduces the bioburden of wounds. In a pilot study, 10 patients were randomly placed in either an experimental VAC group or a saline-gauze control group. A greater reduction in size and faster healing was noted in the VAC-treated group, but it was not statistically significant (3).

Growth Factors

Growth factor therapy, available either in combination through a platelet releasate or through recombinant platelet-derived growth factor (PDGF) technology, has been shown to improve healing of diabetic neuropathic foot ulcers. Regranex (becaplermin; Ortho-McNeil, Raritan, NJ) contains recombinant PDGF and has been studied in several randomized clinical trials with modest improvement in healing (50% healing using PDGF vs. 35% healing using normal saline dressings at 20 weeks) (4). Recently, topical application of epidermal growth factor demonstrated improved healing of diabetic foot ulcers in a dose-dependent fashion. Factors such as nerve and neurotrophic growth factors and improved delivery of growth factors continue to be evaluated.

Hyperbaric Oxygen

Hyperbaric oxygen therapy (HBO) is currently reimbursed by the Center for Medicare and Medicaid Services in the U.S. for the treatment of diabetic foot ulcers, and limited evidence suggests its efficacy for both ischemic and nonischemic ulcers in several small trials (5). One study evaluated 18 diabetic patients with ischemic, nonhealing lower-extremity ulcers randomly assigned to receive either 100% oxygen (treatment group) or air (control group) at 2.4 atmospheres of absolute pressure for 90 min/day (total of 30 treatments). Healing occurred in five of the eight ulcers in the treatment group, compared to one of eight ulcers in the control group, and an associated decrease in wound size was noted ($P = 0.027$). In a study of 28 patients' nonischemic neuropathic diabetic ulcers, a short course of HBO applied twice daily for 5 days a week for 2 weeks resulted in improved transcutaneous oxygen pressure ($tcPO_2$) measurements, and the size of ulcers decreased significantly in the HBO group ($P = 0.03$). However, prolonged benefit was not demonstrated.

Electrical Stimulation

Electrical stimulation appears to increase local blood flow in patients with diabetes (6). In an effort to evaluate the effects of two stimulation waveforms on healing rates in patients with diabetes and open ulcers, 80 patients received daily stimulation with either a biphasic square-wave pulse (asymmetric or symmetric) or a control treatment, which consisted of either very low levels of stimulation current or no electrical stimulation. Asymmetric biphasic stimulation significantly increased healing by nearly 60% over the control group's rate of healing.

Topical Radiant Heat

Topical radiant heat therapy (TRH) is a novel method of modulating the wound environment. It optimizes the enzymatic processes involved in wound healing, which prefer a normothermic environment (most wounds are hypothermic relative to core body temperature). In a study, 20 patients with diabetic foot ulcers were treated with noncontact normothermic wound therapy (Warm-Up; Augustine Medical, Eden Prairie, MN) applied for 1 h, 3 times daily until healing (or 12 weeks), or standard care (saline-moistened gauze applied once a day). Ulcers treated with noncontact normothermic wound therapy (NNWT) had a greater mean percent of wound closure than control-treated ulcers at each evaluation point (weeks 1–12). After 12 weeks, 70% of the wounds treated with NNWT were healed, compared with 40% for the control group.

References

1. Veves A, Falanga V, Armstrong DG, Sabolinski ML, Apligraf Diabetic Foot Ulcer Study: Graftskin, a human skin equivalent, is effective in the management of non-infected neuropathic diabetic foot ulcers: a prospective randomized multicenter clinical trial. *Diabetes Care* 24:290–295, 2001

2. Gentzkow GD, Iwasaki SD, Hershon KS, Mengel M, Prendergast JJ, Ricotta JJ, Steed DP, Lipkin S: Use of Dermagraft, a cultured human dermis, to treat diabetic foot ulcers. *Diabetes Care* 19:350–354, 1996

3. McCallon SK, Knight CA, Valiulus JP, Cunningham MW, McCulloch JM, Farinas LP: Vacuum-assisted closure versus saline-moistened gauze in the healing of postoperative diabetic foot wounds. *Ostomy Wound Manage* 46:28–32, 34, 2000

4. Steed DL: Clinical evaluation of recombinant human platelet-derived growth factor for the treatment of lower extremity diabetic ulcers. Diabetic Ulcer Study Group. *J Vasc Surg* 21:71–78, 1995

5. Kranke P, Bennett M, Roeckl-Wiedmann I, Debus S: Hyperbaric oxygen therapy for chronic wounds. *Cochrane Database Syst Rev* 2:CD004123, 2004

6. Baker LL, Chambers R, DeMuth SK, Villar F: Effects of electrical stimulation on wound healing in patients with diabetic ulcers. *Diabetes Care* 20:405–412, 1997

9

The Diabetic Charcot Foot: Recognition, Evaluation, and Management

Lee J. Sanders, DPM
Robert G. Frykberg, DPM, MPH

DIABETES IS THE LEADING CAUSE of neuropathic osteo-arthropathy (Charcot's joint disease, Charcot foot), a potentially disabling condition affecting the foot and ankle. Jean-Martin Charcot and Charles Féré published the first scientific investigation of this condition, which affects the short bones and small joints of the tabetic foot, in 1883 (1). Until that time, nearly all published observations of neuropathic bone and joint lesions concerned the long bones of the limbs and their large articulations (1,2).

Symptoms

Early symptoms of the Charcot foot can be subtle, with mild swelling, redness, and a localized increase in the skin temperature of the foot and ankle, so the condition often goes unrecognized. Sometimes the foot suddenly and unexpectedly collapses, with fractures, dislocations, and ulceration. Remarkably, these destructive events occur in the absence of major trauma. Even after the condition has matured, the bone and joint changes may resemble osteomyelitis, further confusing the diagnosis.

Unfortunately, recognition and treatment of the Charcot foot remain significant problems, and the precise pathogenesis of the condition is an enigma. Clinicians must therefore be watchful for it, especially in that subset of diabetic patients who are considered to be at high risk for developing the condition. These patients typically have a long history of diabetes (10–15 years' duration), are in their sixth decade of life (those with type 1 diabetes could be younger), and demonstrate evidence of sensory-motor-autonomic neuropathy. The clinical picture is characterized by loss of protective sensation, lack of deep tendon reflexes, diminished or absent vibratory sensation, and the presence of palpable (often bounding) pedal pulses. Prior to the acute onset of neuropathic osteoarthropathy, patients may experience painful sensory neuropathy characterized by lancinating pains, like a shower of electric needles, of short duration but recurrent throughout the day (3–5). Characteristics include the following (3–6):

- Acute Charcot foot may mimic cellulitis, acute gouty arthritis, or thrombophlebitis. Early on, it may be indistinguishable from osteoarthritis or infection.
- Pain may be absent or minimal—which is astonishing, considering the extensive bone and joint pathology seen in some cases.
- Radiographs may initially appear unremarkable. Early radiographic findings can be absent or so subtle that they are easily missed by the untrained eye. A minimally displaced fracture at the base of the second metatarsal, which may precede collapse of the tarsometatarsal joints (Fig. 9.1), is especially likely to be missed. A negative report can lead the clinician to mistakenly treat the condition as an infection, gout, or deep vein thrombosis and to lose valuable time. (This error can also become a litigious issue for the clinician and the radiologist.) Whenever possible, clinicians should view the radiographs themselves and not rely solely on the radiologist's interpretation.
- Early identification of Charcot's joint disease is crucial, with immediate rest, immobilization, and off-loading recommended. Until the diagnosis of Charcot foot can be safely

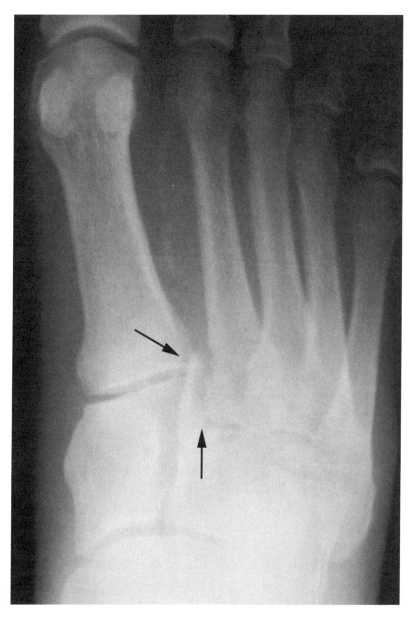

Figure 9.1 Early presentation of the Charcot foot with subtle findings at the tarsometatarsal joints (pattern II). Note the displaced fracture at the base of the second metatarsal bone with >2 mm separation at the bases of the first and second metatarsal bones.

ruled out, err on the side of conservative treatment, with immobilization and off-loading. A cavalier, watch-and-wait approach could be disastrous.

■ For those at high risk, patient education is critical. Discuss the implications of sensory loss, the signs and symptoms of Charcot's joint disease, the importance of therapeutic footwear, and the need for preventive foot care.

Prevalence and Risk Factors

The prevalence of diagnosed neuropathic osteoarthropathy associated with diabetes mellitus has been reported to be from 0.08% to 7.5% (3,5). A study of radiographic abnormalities in the feet of neuropathic diabetic subjects revealed that 9% of the patients had evidence of Charcot's joint disease (7). The true incidence of osteoarthropathy in diabetes is limited by few prospective or population-based studies. Available data are mainly based on retrospective studies of small single-center cohorts. In addition, because many cases go undetected, especially in the early stages, the prevalence has probably been under-estimated. However, reported cases of the diabetic Charcot foot appear to be on the rise as a result of increased awareness of its signs and symptoms.

The primary risk factors for the Charcot foot are the presence of dense peripheral sensory neuropathy, palpable pedal pulses, and a history of preceding trauma, often minor in nature. A careful history will often reveal a precipitating event, such as a minor ankle sprain or contusion that preceded collapse of the foot. Foot and ankle deformities, limited joint mobility (such as limited ankle joint dorsiflexion caused by contracture of the Achilles tendon), faulty biomechanics, or surgical trauma can also trigger Charcot's joint disease (3–5).

Clinicians must be aware that the Charcot foot is a progressive condition characterized by joint dislocation, pathologic fractures, and collapse of the foot and ankle. Ultimately, this condition can lead to debilitating deformity, instability of the foot and ankle, ulceration, infection, and amputation.

Etiology of Neuropathic Osteoarthropathy

Charcot's joint disease is most likely the result of the combined effects of neurovascular and neurotraumatic etiologies (2–5,8). Minor injury of a neuropathic limb can precipitate the development of an acute Charcot foot. Autonomic nervous system dysfunction has also been associated with neuropathic osteoarthropathy.

A neurally initiated vascular reflex leading to increased peripheral blood flow and active bone resorption may be another important etiologic factor. Autonomic neuropathy with loss of vasomotor control and increased peripheral blood flow to the bone, coupled with an inflammatory hyperemia of the soft tissues, results in resorption and weakening of bone. Atrophic osteopenic bone is easily fractured or fragmented. Sensory neuropathy renders the patient unaware of precipitating injuries and the osseous destruction taking place during unrestricted physical activities. A vicious cycle develops in which the patient continues to walk on the injured foot, thereby causing further damage.

Diagnosis of the Acute Charcot Foot

Diagnosis of the acute Charcot foot is based on the following findings: unilateral swelling of the foot or ankle, elevated skin temperature compared to the contralateral limb, erythema, peripheral neuropathy, and variable radiographic changes. As previously mentioned, early radiographic findings may be negative. Positive findings may reveal bone resorption (typically in the forefoot), diastasis (>2 mm separation at the bases of the first and second metatarsal bone), subluxation/dislocation (typically at the tarsometatarsal, naviculocuneiform, or midtarsal joints), or fracture(s). Look carefully at the base of the second metatarsal (Fig. 9.1).

Radiographs of the opposite foot are helpful for comparison. Bilateral involvement has been reported to occur in 5.9–39.3% of cases. Usually, no further imaging studies are needed to establish the diagnosis.

The presence of ulceration may further complicate the diagnosis, making it difficult to differentiate between acute Charcot's neuropathic osteoarthropathy and osteomyelitis; additional laboratory studies may help. The white blood cell count is typically not elevated in patients with neuropathic osteoarthropathy, but the erythrocyte sedimentation rate may be mildly elevated. Ulcers that probe to bone are highly suggestive of osteomyelitis.

A bone biopsy, when indicated, is the most specific test to distinguish between osteomyelitis and osteoarthropathy. Characteristic histologic findings associated with neuropathic osteoarthropathy include the following:

- erosion of articular cartilage
- active resorption of bone with thin, widely spaced trabeculae
- increased vascularity
- new bone formation
- remodeling

When the ankle joint is involved, there is a striking pathologic feature of bone and cartilage debris (detritus) ground into the synovial tissue and articular cartilage (3).

Technetium bone scans are limited in differentiating osteomyelitis from acute Charcot's neuropathic osteoarthropathy because increased uptake on delayed images is seen in patients with neuropathic noninfective bone disease as well as in those with osteomyelitis. Indium-111 WBC imaging is more specific, with high negative predictive value for osteomyelitis. Additional diagnostic studies that may help differentiate Charcot's arthropathy from osteomyelitis include bone scans utilizing WBCs labeled with Tc-HMPAO and magnetic resonance imaging (3).

Classification of the Charcot Foot

The most commonly referenced classification of Charcot's arthropathy is based on radiographic findings associated with stages of the disease process. The Eichenholtz classification divides the disease into three radiographically distinct stages: development, coalescence, and reconstruction (9). The development stage represents the acute destructive phase of this disease and is characterized by soft tissue swelling, intra-articular fractures, osteochondral fragmentation, or joint dislocation. The coalescence stage represents the reparative phase of healing and is marked by a reduction in soft tissue swelling, bone callus proliferation, consolidation of bony fragments, and healing of fractures. Finally, the reconstruction stage reflects further repair and remodeling of bone and is evidenced by bony ankylosis and hypertrophic proliferation.

Eichenholtz's radiographic classification is descriptive, but it has limited clinical value. In practice, the stage of development is considered active, whereas the stages of coalescence and reconstruction are quiescent or reparative. This classification fails to identify the earliest presentation of the Charcot foot (prior to the development of radiographic evidence), the location involved, and association with ulcers.

A more recent descriptive classification of the Charcot foot is based on anatomical patterns of bone and joint destruction. Although this approach to classification does not indicate the stage or activity of disease, it more precisely identifies anatomic sites of involvement and the association of foot deformity with plantar ulceration. Five characteristic patterns (Fig. 9.2) range from the forefoot (pattern I), to the tarsometatarsal joints (pattern II), the lesser tarsus (pattern III), the ankle and subtalar joints (pattern IV), and the posterior calcaneus (pattern V). Patterns I and II are associated with deformity and ulceration. Joint involvement is most frequently seen in patterns I, II, and III, and the most severe structural deformity and functional instability are associated with patterns II and IV (3,5,10).

Management of the Charcot Foot

Management of the Charcot foot is determined by the acuteness of symptoms (acute vs. chronic), the anatomical pattern of bone and joint involvement, and the degree of involvement (such as deformity, fractures, fragmentation of bone, and instability), as well as the presence of ulceration and wound infection. Immobilization and reduction of weight-bearing stress are the foundations of treatment for acute Charcot foot. Most Charcot foot experts recommend no weight bearing on the affected extremity. Off-loading the foot effectively reduces pressure, but this strategy may increase stress on the

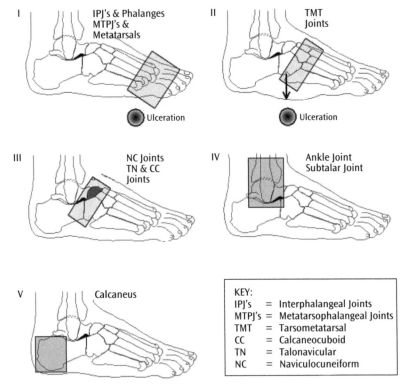

Figure 9.2 Five anatomical patterns of bone and joint involvement commonly reported in patients with diabetic neuropathic osteoarthropathy (Charcot's joint disease). *From* Sanders and Frykberg, p. 308, reproduced with permission (5).

contralateral limb, precipitating neuropathic fractures and ulceration on the previously unaffected foot.

Reduced skin temperature and swelling are markers of healing. At this point, protected weight bearing is permitted, usually with a total contact cast, walking brace, or patellar tendon-bearing orthosis. Patients can then ambulate safely while bony consolidation and remodeling take place. Mean treatment time (casting followed by removable cast walker) before the return to therapeutic footwear is approximately 4–6 months.

Other treatments under investigation include pharmacologic therapy of the Charcot foot with bisphosphonates to inhibit osteoclastic activity (11). Similarly, managing acute cases with ancillary bone stimulators to promote more rapid consolidation of fractures has been explored (12). Although promising, neither of these adjunctive treatments has been conclusively proved effective through large, prospective, randomized clinical trials.

Surgical Management

Surgery should be considered when deformity or instability of the foot cannot be accommodated or controlled by prescription footwear or bracing. Advances in surgical techniques have improved outcomes; however, complication rates are still high. Surgical approaches to treatment range from simple ostectomy to major reconstruction of the foot with open-reduction and internal fixation of fractures and dislocations. Interest has been growing in applying external fixation devices (frames) to correct and maintain a plantigrade position of the foot during healing. A clinical practice pathway summarizing the diagnostic and treatment considerations for the diabetic Charcot foot is illustrated in Fig. 9.3 (13).

Summary

Charcot's joint disease of the foot and ankle is a serious complication of diabetes that is, unfortunately, frequently overlooked and often debilitating. Diagnosis is made based on clinical suspicion of the disorder in high-risk patients. Successful treatment hinges on early recognition, immobilization, and off-loading until inflammation has subsided and the foot is stable. Therapeutic footwear and bracing are integral components of treatment. Medical management of the Charcot foot remains the standard of care for most patients, with surgical intervention reserved for the most difficult cases. Pharmacologic treatment to inhibit osteoclastic activity and shorten the course of the disease is under investigation.

Nevertheless, primary prevention of the Charcot foot should be our objective. Patient and physician education regarding foot inspection, risk factors, and metabolic control of diabetes, as well as pharmacotherapy for the prevention of peripheral neuropathy, may facilitate this goal.

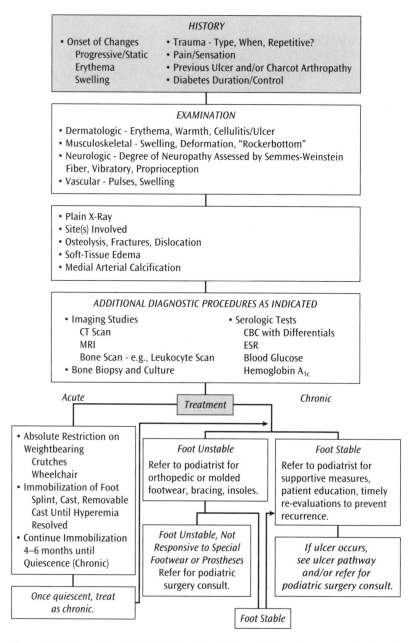

HISTORY

- Onset of Changes
  - Progressive/Static
  - Erythema
  - Swelling
- Trauma - Type, When, Repetitive?
- Pain/Sensation
- Previous Ulcer and/or Charcot Arthropathy
- Diabetes Duration/Control

EXAMINATION

- Dermatologic - Erythema, Warmth, Cellulitis/Ulcer
- Musculoskeletal - Swelling, Deformation, "Rockerbottom"
- Neurologic - Degree of Neuropathy Assessed by Semmes-Weinstein Fiber, Vibratory, Proprioception
- Vascular - Pulses, Swelling

- Plain X-Ray
- Site(s) Involved
- Osteolysis, Fractures, Dislocation
- Soft-Tissue Edema
- Medial Arterial Calcification

ADDITIONAL DIAGNOSTIC PROCEDURES AS INDICATED

- Imaging Studies
  - CT Scan
  - MRI
  - Bone Scan - e.g., Leukocyte Scan
- Bone Biopsy and Culture
- Serologic Tests
  - CBC with Differentials
  - ESR
  - Blood Glucose
  - Hemoglobin A_{1c}

Acute   **Treatment**   *Chronic*

- Absolute Restriction on Weightbearing
  - Crutches
  - Wheelchair
- Immobilization of Foot Splint, Cast, Removable Cast Until Hyperemia Resolved
- Continue Immobilization 4–6 months until Quiescence (Chronic)

Once quiescent, treat as chronic.

Foot Unstable

Refer to podiatrist for orthopedic or molded footwear, bracing, insoles.

Foot Unstable, Not Responsive to Special Footwear or Prostheses Refer for podiatric surgery consult.

Foot Stable

Refer to podiatrist for supportive measures, patient education, timely re-evaluations to prevent recurrence.

If ulcer occurs, see ulcer pathway and/or refer for podiatric surgery consult.

Foot Stable

Figure 9.3 Charcot Foot: A Clinical Practice Pathway. This pathway was developed by the Core Clinical Practice Committee of the American College of Foot and Ankle Surgeons (ACFAS) and is based on current clinical practice and extensive review of the literature. *From* Frykberg et al., reproduced with permission (13).

References

1. Charcot JM, Féré C: Affections osseuses et articulaires du pied chez les tabétiques (Pied tabétique). *Archives de Neurologie* 6:305–319, 1883

2. Sanders LJ: The Charcot foot: historical perspective, 1827–2003. *Diabetes Metab Res Rev* 20 (Suppl. 1):S4–S8, 2004

3. Sanders LJ, Frykberg RG: Charcot neuroarthropathy of the foot. In Levin and O'Neal's *The Diabetic Foot.* 6th ed. Bowker JH, Pfeifer MA, Eds. St. Louis, Mosby Year Book, 2001, p. 439

4. Frykberg RG, Kozak GP: The diabetic Charcot foot. In *Management of Diabetic Foot Problems.* 2nd ed. Kozak GP, Campbell DR, Frykberg RG, Habershaw GM, Eds. Philadelphia, WB Saunders, 1995, p. 88–97

5. Sanders LJ, Frykberg RG: Diabetic neuropathic osteoarthropathy: the Charcot foot. In *The High Risk Foot in Diabetes Mellitus.* Frykberg RG, Ed. New York, Churchill Livingstone, 1991, p. 297

6. Caputo GM, Ulbrecht J, Cavanagh PR, Juliano P: The Charcot foot in diabetes: six key points. *Am Fam Physician* 57:2705–2710, 1998

7. Cavanagh PR, Young MJ, Adams JE, Vickers KL, Boulton AJ: Radiographic abnormalities in the feet of patients with diabetic neuropathy. *Diabetes Care* 17:201–209, 1994

8. Brower AC, Allman RM: Pathogenesis of the neurotrophic joint: neurotraumatic vs. neurovascular. *Radiology* 139:349–354, 1981

9. Eichenholtz SN: *Charcot Joints.* Springfield, IL, Charles C. Thomas, 1966

10. Sanders LJ, Mrdjenovich D: Anatomical patterns of bone and joint destruction in neuropathic diabetics (Abstract). *Diabetes* 40 (Suppl. 1):529A, 1991

11. Jude EB, Selby PL, Burgess J, Lilleystone P, Mawer EB, Page SR, Donohoe M, Foster AV, Edmonds ME, Boulton AJ: Bisphosphonates in the treatment of Charcot neuroarthropathy: a double-blind randomised controlled trial. *Diabetologia* 44:2032–2037, 2001

12. Hanft JR, Goggin JP, Landsman A, Surprenant M: The role of combined magnetic field bone growth stimulation as an adjunct in the treatment of neuroarthropathy/Charcot joint: an expanded pilot study. *J Foot Ankle Surg* 37:510–515, 1998

13. Frykberg RG, Armstrong DG, Giurini J, Edwards A, Kravette M, Kravitz S, Ross C, Stavosky J, Stuck R, Vanore J: Diabetic foot disorders: a clinical practice guideline. *J Foot Ankle Surg* 39 (Suppl. 1):1–60, 2000

10

Infection in the Diabetic Foot

Anthony R. Berendt, BM, BCh, MA, FRCP
Benjamin A. Lipsky, MD, FACP

A FOOT INFECTION IS one of the most common clinical events leading to lower-limb amputation in people with diabetes (1). Infection generally begins in an ulceration, which is why prevention and treatment of foot ulcers are so important (2). These infections must be addressed promptly and effectively, as delay increases the risk of soft tissue loss, bone involvement, and poor outcome. Uncertainties persist on many issues, but two international committees have recently produced consensus guidelines that offer a framework for assessing and treating diabetic foot infections (3–5).

Epidemiology

Foot ulceration is the major risk factor for infection, but only ~40–80% of ulcers eventually become infected. Peripheral arterial disease and perhaps other comorbidities, such as suboptimal glycemic control, appear to increase the risk of infection. Approximately one-fifth of infections involve bone (osteomyelitis), and about one-third are classified as severe. Infection dramatically increases the risk of hospitalization and amputation.

Definitions

Understanding the relationship between pathogenic bacteria and the human host is essential in formulating infection management strategies (6):

- **Contamination** of a wound occurs when nonresident bacteria are externally introduced to host tissue. The number and virulence of the organisms and the robustness of the host's immune system determine the next steps.
- **Colonization** occurs when new bacteria introduced into an ulcer replicate and establish a physiological state of coexistence without overt tissue damage or host response.
- **Infection** is diagnosed when either contaminating or colonizing microorganisms invade host tissue, inciting an inflammatory response and causing cellular damage.
- **Diabetic foot infection** refers to infections below the malleoli in a person with diabetes. Any type of trauma that disrupts the protective skin envelope can lead to an infection.

Diagnosis

Because bacteria can be isolated from both colonized and infected tissues, microbiological tests can be used to diagnose infection only when samples are taken from sites that have no resident flora (i.e., deep, viable tissues) by methods that avoid contamination during sampling. Microbiology is useful to identify the causative pathogens (and their antibiotic susceptibilities) in clinically infected wounds.

The clinical diagnosis of infection requires evidence of host tissue damage and response. Consensus criteria for diagnosing infection are the presence of two or more of the following:

- erythema (>0.5 cm from the ulcer margin)
- local swelling or induration
- local warmth
- local tenderness or pain
- purulent discharge

Other possible signs of infection are when the wound fails to heal as expected, the quantity or character of ulcer drainage changes, or a foul smell or wound necrosis develops.

Clinical Manifestations and Classification

Types of infection range from paronychia (a complication of ingrown toenails) to infections of ulcers, deep soft tissue compartments, fascial planes, tendon sheaths, joints, and bones. Because anatomic schemes are inadequate to establish priorities for clinical management, the consensus groups classified infections according to severity:

- *Uninfected ulcers* do not meet the criteria outlined above for the clinical diagnosis of infection. They usually pose no immediate threat to limb or patient.
- *Mild infections* involve only the skin and superficial subcutaneous tissue. Any erythema extends ≤2 cm from the ulcer margin and any necrosis is minimal. These infections pose minimal immediate risk.
- *Moderate infections* are a heterogeneous group. They include those in which erythema extends >2 cm beyond the ulcer border or ulcers in which infection breaches the superficial fascia and so involves deeper structures, including tendon, bone, or joint. There may be deep abscess formation, necrosis, and gangrene. Such infections often pose immediate risk to the foot.
- *Severe infections* are clinically similar to moderate ones in anatomic extent, but the patient manifests a systemic inflammatory response in the form of fever, leukocytosis, hypotension, or marked metabolic derangement. Because these responses are often muted in people with long-standing diabetes, their presence suggests more serious disease, including complicating bacteremia. Severe infections can pose immediate threat to life and limb.

These classification schemes correspond directly to Grades 0 (uninfected) to 4 (severe) of the diabetic foot ulcer classification scheme recently produced for research purposes by international consensus (3). This scheme considers **p**erfusion, **e**xtent of ulcer (area), **d**epth of wound, **i**nfection, and **s**ensation (making the acronym PEDIS) to categorize the case mix of ulcers studied in trials.

Assessment

Optimal treatment of the infection requires carefully considering not only the foot, but also the person to whom it is (and hopefully will remain) attached. The clinician must assess

- *The patient:* systemic features, cognitive function, psychosocial situation, understanding of and engagement with their own health, availability of other caregivers
- *The limb:* arterial perfusion, extent of infection (if spreading cellulitis/fasciitis)
- *The foot:* biomechanics, neuropathy, ischemia, evidence of deep space infections or extensive soft tissue involvement, bony damage
- *The ulcer:* extent, depth, necrosis, involvement of bone, joint, or tendon

Assessing the wound may require some debridement of callus, ulcer slough, and necrotic tissue. If a sterile blunt metal probe introduced into the ulcer strikes rock-hard, gritty material (a positive "probe to bone" test), there is a moderate likelihood of osteomyelitis (7). Probing can also reveal loose bony fragments, foreign bodies in the ulcer, and communication into joints or deep spaces. Plain X-rays of the foot are adequate for most infected lesions; if the patient could have other bony disorders (such as Charcot foot) or it is important to know the extent of the soft tissue infection, consider magnetic resonance imaging. A complete blood count and inflammatory markers (erythrocyte sedimentation rate or C-reactive protein) may help assess the severity of the infection. For most moderate and virtually all severe infections, an experienced surgeon should assess the patient to determine whether surgery is needed.

Microbiological Diagnosis

Uninfected ulcers need not be cultured, and many acute and antibiotic-naïve mild infections do not require microbiological sampling, as the pathogens are overwhelmingly aerobic gram-positive cocci—that is, *Staphylococcus aureus* and beta-hemolytic streptococci (8). Specimens must be cultured, however, when the infection is extensive, empiric treatment is failing, or antibiotic resistance (e.g., methicillin-resistant *S. aureus*) is a concern. Obtain specimens by aspiration of pus, curettage of the debrided ulcer base (not of slough), or deeper tissue biopsy in preference to wound swabs. Clearly identifying the type of specimen and communicating with the laboratory will optimize processing and analysis of the samples.

Treatment Planning

After assessing the severity of the infection and its key accompanying features, the clinician is ready to formulate a treatment plan (9). Treatment could include debriding, off-loading pressure, correcting severe ischemia if present, draining any abscesses, removing necrotic tissue, and correcting systemic disturbances such as electrolyte imbalance or hyperglycemia. The following will help the clinician choose the venue for care (ambulatory versus hospital) and an appropriate empiric antibiotic regimen (10).

- *Uninfected ulcers* do not require antibiotic therapy, because it has not been shown to improve ulcer healing or prevent infection (11).
- *Mild infections* can be treated on an ambulatory basis, unless the patient has cognitive or social impairments affecting his or her ability to care for the ulcer and follow antibiotic therapy. Semisynthetic penicillins (dicloxacillin, cloxacillin, flucloxacillin), or first-generation cephalosporins (e.g., cephalexin) are usually adequate for first-line treatment.
- *Moderate infections* needing urgent empiric antibiotic therapy require a relatively broad-spectrum coverage, including gram-positive cocci, as well as aerobic gram-negative rods and anaer-

obes. The latter organisms are more frequent in chronic and complex infections, which are often those that have failed prior antibiotic therapy. Appropriate choices include combinations of a fluoroquinolone (e.g., ciprofloxacin or levofloxacin) with clindamycin or a penicillin/penicillinase inhibitor (e.g., ampicillin-sulbactam or amoxicillin-clavulanate). Hospitalization may be required for surgical intervention or, occasionally, for special diagnostic tests. For moderate infections that are chronic (e.g., osteomyelitis), it is often better to hold antibiotic therapy until proper cultures are obtained and processed.

■ *Severe infections* must always be treated urgently, with initial hospitalization and intravenous antibiotics. The selected antimicrobial regimen should cover the above-cited organisms as well as *Pseudomonas aeruginosa* and other resistant aerobic gram-negative rods. Appropriate regimens include carbapenems (e.g., imipenem-cilastatin) or antipseudomonal penicillins with a beta-lactamase inhibitor (e.g., piperacillin-tazobactam). Always consider the potential need for surgery, in addition to the medical treatment.

Osteomyelitis

Diagnosing and treating osteomyelitis are particularly difficult (12,13). Noninfectious neuropathic osteoarthropathy, which causes changes on plain radiography that can mimic infection, is frequently present in those with long-standing diabetes. Most radionuclide isotope scans are insufficiently sensitive and specific to distinguish between the two conditions, although modern forms of white-cell labeling show promise (14,15). Magnetic resonance imaging currently offers the most accurate diagnosis when properly interpreted (16–18).

Treatment of osteomyelitis traditionally requires both surgical resection of infected or necrotic bone and prolonged intravenous antibiotics. The advent of highly bioavailable oral antibiotics has substantially reduced or eliminated the period of intravenous therapy. In several retrospective reviews, diabetic foot osteomyelitis was arrested without surgery in 60–70% of patients, but randomized comparisons of early surgery versus antibiotics alone are needed (19).

Duration of Therapy

The severity of infection and the presence of bony involvement largely determine the length of treatment. If the infection does not respond as expected, reassess the patient's adherence to the antibiotic (and ulcer care) regimen and check for any undetected abscess, necrosis, or ischemia. Recommended durations of therapy are as follows:

- **Mild infections:** 1–2 weeks, usually
- **Moderate infections:** often 2–4 weeks (if no bone involvement)
- **Severe infections:** 2–4 weeks, depending on the nature of any surgery and the presence of bacteremia
- **Osteomyelitis:** Duration depends on the extent of residual bone involvement after any surgical intervention:

  - All involved bone is removed (ablative surgery): treatment based on soft tissue involvement; if uninfected, prophylax for up to 72 h; if infected, treat for 2 weeks
  - Infected but viable bone remains: 4–6 weeks
  - Dead bone remains: minimum of 6–12 weeks. Long-term antibiotic regimens are sometimes used to suppress, rather than attempt to cure, infection.

Summary

To help avoid encouraging antibiotic resistance, the length and breadth of antibiotic therapy should be tailored to the severity of the infection; choose the narrowest spectrum and shortest duration appropriate. If treatment fails or progress is slow, reevaluate the wound as well as the patient, rather than reflexively adding additional agents. Future studies need to establish the most cost-effective diagnostic and treatment strategies, especially in relation to osteomyelitis.

References

1. Reiber GE, Pecoraro RE, Koepsell TD: Risk factors for amputation in patients with diabetes mellitus: a case-control study. *Ann Intern Med* 117:97–105, 1992

2. Boulton AJ, Kirsner RS, Vileikyte L: Clinical practice. Neuropathic diabetic foot ulcers. *N Engl J Med* 351:48–55, 2004

3. International Working Group on the Diabetic Foot: *International Consensus on the Diabetic Foot.* CD-ROM. Amsterdam, Netherlands, International Diabetes Federation, 2003. Web site: http://www.idf.org/bookshop

4. Lipsky BA: A report from the international consensus on diagnosing and treating the infected diabetic foot. *Diabetes Metab Res Rev* 20 (Suppl. 1):S68–S77, 2004

5. Lipsky BA, Berendt AR, Deery HG 2nd, Embil JM, Joseph WS, Karchmer AW, LeFrock J, Lew DP, Mader JT, Norden C, Tan JS: IDSA Guideline: diagnosis and treatment of diabetic foot infections. *Clin Infect Dis* 39:885–910, 2004

6. Lipsky BA, Berendt AR: Principles and practice of antibiotic therapy of diabetic foot infections. *Diabetes Metab Res Rev* 16 (Suppl. 1):S42–S46, 2000

7. Grayson ML, Gibbons GW, Balogh K, Levin E, Karchmer AW: Probing to bone in infected pedal ulcers: a clinical sign of underlying osteomyelitis in diabetic patients. *JAMA* 273:721–723, 1995

8. Lipsky BA, Pecoraro RE, Wheat LJ: The diabetic foot: soft tissue and bone infection. *Infect Dis Clin North Am* 4:409–432, 1990

9. Lipsky BA, Berendt AR, Embil J, De Lalla F: Diagnosing and treating diabetic foot infections. *Diabetes Metab Res Rev* 20 (Suppl. 1):S56–S64, 2004

10. Lipsky BA: Evidence-based antibiotic therapy of diabetic foot infections. *FEMS Immunol Med Microbiol* 26:267–276, 1999

11. Berendt AR, Lipsky BA: Should antibiotics be used in the treatment of the diabetic foot? *The Diabetic Foot* 6:18–28, 2003

12. Lipsky BA: Osteomyelitis of the foot in diabetic patients. *Clin Infect Dis* 25:1318–1326, 1997

13. Berendt AR, Lipsky BA: Bone and joint infections in the diabetic foot. *Current Treatment Options in Infectious Diseases* 5:345–360, 2003

14. Sella EJ, Grosser DM: Imaging modalities of the diabetic foot. *Clin Podiatr Med Surg* 20:729–740, 2003

15. Hakki S, Harwood SJ, Morrissey MA, Camblin JG, Laven DL, Webster WB Jr: Comparative study of monoclonal antibody scan in diagnosing orthopaedic infection. *Clin Orthop* 275–285, 1997

16. Greenspan A, Stadalnik RC: A musculoskeletal radiologist's view of nuclear medicine. *Semin Nucl Med* 27:372–385, 1997

17. Ledermann HP, Morrison WB, Schweitzer ME: MR image analysis of pedal osteomyelitis: distribution, patterns of spread, and frequency of associated ulceration and septic arthritis. *Radiology* 223:747–755, 2002

18. Schweitzer ME, Morrison WB: MR imaging of the diabetic foot. *Radiol Clin North Am* 42:61–71, 2004

19. Jeffcoate WJ, Lipsky BA: Controversies in diagnosing and managing osteomyelitis of the foot in diabetes. *Clin Infect Dis* 39 (Suppl. 2):S115–S122, 2004

11

Evaluation and Management of Peripheral Arterial Disease

Joseph L. Mills, Sr., MD

FOR THE 18 MILLION INDIVIDUALS with diabetes mellitus in the United States, foot problems—ulceration, infection, and ischemia—are a major cause of hospitalization. Most of these problems are a result of neuropathy and superimposed infection, but peripheral arterial disease (PAD) is an important contributing factor in 10–30% of cases (1,2). The annual health care cost for these foot problems exceeds $1 billion (3).

Arteriosclerosis Obliterans

Serial clinical studies have noted the development of arteriosclerosis obliterans (ASO) in 50% of patients with type 2 diabetes within 15 years of disease onset (4); the prevalence of ASO is 12–28 times greater than that observed in age- and sex-matched control groups (5). Additional risk factors that are associated with increased prevalence as well as progression of ASO in patients with type 2 diabetes include cigarette smoking, having diabetes for >10 years, HDL cholesterol <40 mg/dl, systolic blood pressure >145 mmHg, and obesity index >2.83 g/cm (3,6–8).

Myths about ASO

Several myths about ASO or PAD in diabetic patients are pervasive in the medical and patient communities and need to be dispelled. ASO in patients with diabetes mellitus is histologically indistinguishable from that of individuals without diabetes (9). The major and clinically important difference is disease distribution. In those without diabetes, proximal arterial occlusive disease (aorto-iliac segments and distal superficial femoral artery) is more common, whereas in diabetic patients, ASO commonly affects the deep femoral artery and the medium-sized, below-knee popliteal and tibio-peroneal arteries (infrageniculate vessels).

Diabetic patients sometimes present with foot lesions, palpable femoral and popliteal pulses, and absent foot pulses, but the cause is not microvascular disease, but ASO in the infrageniculate, or "trifurcation," vessels. The distal peroneal, dorsal pedal, and digital arteries are frequently spared, and the peroneal and pedal vessels are often sites for bypass graft insertion.

There remains a widespread misconception that patients with diabetes mellitus have arteriolar occlusive disease that can cause pedal ischemia and gangrene, even in the presence of palpable pedal pulses. The myth of a unique "diabetic microangiopathy" stems from a single amputation study reported in 1959 that demonstrated periodic acid–Schiff (PAS) positive material in the arterioles of diabetic patients who had undergone major limb amputation (10). Subsequent detailed angiographic, physiologic, and histologic studies have not confirmed the presence of a unique diabetic microangiopathy (3,4,9).

Although studies have confirmed that patients with diabetes have an abnormal, thickened basement membrane in the capillaries, the membrane does not appear to be associated with gangrene (3). In fact, despite this abnormality, the patency and limb salvage results of lower-extremity bypass in patients with diabetes are equivalent to those without diabetes (11), with the exception of individuals with end-stage renal disease (12). This observation argues strongly against the presence of clinically significant "small-vessel disease" or microangiopathy.

Treating Infection

Management of neuropathy (through off-loading, callus debridement, and proper footwear) and infection (through appropriate antibiotics and surgical debridement) is discussed elsewhere in this book and is critical to preventing major limb amputation. Infection should be promptly and aggressively treated; wide, open debridements are frequently needed to drain purulence and remove necrotic tissue. Assessing the vascularity of every patient presenting with foot ulceration, infection, or frank gangrene and promptly recognizing and quantifying ischemia are essential. Repeated debridement of a nonhealing ischemic foot is clinically unacceptable and destined to result in major limb amputation.

Pulse Palpation and Other Noninvasive Tests

The most important component of the physical examination, from a vascular surgeon's standpoint, is peripheral pulse palpation. The presence of clearly palpable dorsal pedal and posterior tibial pulses usually indicates adequate circulation; sufficient debridement and control of infection heals 90% of cases.

All patients lacking palpable foot pulses should undergo noninvasive testing such as Doppler-derived ankle pressure measurement and ankle-brachial index determination, digital or toe pressure measurements, and pulse volume recordings (PVRs). Unfortunately, due to extensive medial calcification, pedal pulses may not be palpable in some individuals with diabetes (10–20%), and ankle-pressure measurements may also be unreliable if the calcification is severe enough to preclude arterial compression by the cuff (resulting in suprasystolic pressures). Because the digital arteries are often spared, digital waveform and pressure measurements can be useful— we routinely perform them on all patients with foot problems and diabetes. PVRs are helpful because they are unaffected by the presence of arterial wall calcification. Diabetic patients with an absolute ankle pressure <90 mmHg and toe pressures <55 mmHg are unlikely to heal without revascularization (13).

Surgical Options

Patients without foot pulses, with abnormal noninvasive studies, or who fail to heal despite having a foot pulse should be referred to a vascular surgeon. Subsets of patients may have hemodynamically significant tibial artery occlusive disease, despite the presence of a foot pulse, and other individuals, particularly those with end-stage renal disease and heel ulcers, may have regional ischemia of the forefoot or hindfoot (14) that can be corrected by angioplasty, if focal, or by bypass, if more diffuse.

If noninvasive tests indicate ischemia or if healing fails despite proper drainage and debridement, arteriography should be performed by an experienced endovascular surgeon or interventional radiologist. Detailed views of the infrageniculate circulation and magnified views of the foot in at least two projections, especially the lateral one, are essential. Because the peroneal, dorsal pedal, and plantar arteries are usually spared, they are most likely to serve as the recipient artery for a bypass (Figs. 11.1 and 11.2). Many of our colleagues confirm that in limb salvage situations, bypass to the infrageniculate popliteal artery, the tibial arteries, or a pedal or plantar artery is more likely in diabetic individuals (15–18). Except for the insertion site dictated by the more distal distribution pattern, the revascularization procedure does not differ significantly from that performed in individuals without diabetes.

If detailed angiography is performed, >97% of patients threatened with loss of limb who have not previously undergone lower-extremity bypass will be found to have reconstructible arterial disease. In nearly every case, autogenous vein grafts—preferably using the long saphenous, or even the short saphenous, or arm, veins—should be used. Vein graft patency in those with diabetes is equivalent to that of patients without diabetes. The myth of poor results following bypass for patients with diabetes is untrue. In fact, some experienced surgeons report that patency rates for lower-extremity bypass in patients with diabetes exceed those of patients without the condition (11,17).

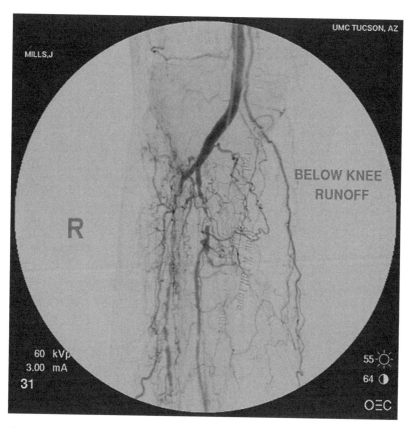

Figure 11.1 Antegrade right femoral diagnostic arteriogram (view at knee level) of an 80-year-old diabetic man with third toe gangrene, a palpable popliteal pulse, absent foot pulses, suprasystolic ankle pressures, and a great toe systolic pressure of 20 mmHg. The popliteal trifurcation is occluded, a common finding in patients with diabetes.

Summary

Patients with diabetes are 20 times more likely to have lower-extremity ASO than individuals without diabetes and 60 times more likely to develop lower-extremity gangrene (3). One-half to two-thirds of major limb amputations in the United States are performed on patients with diabetes. Many of these amputations are the direct

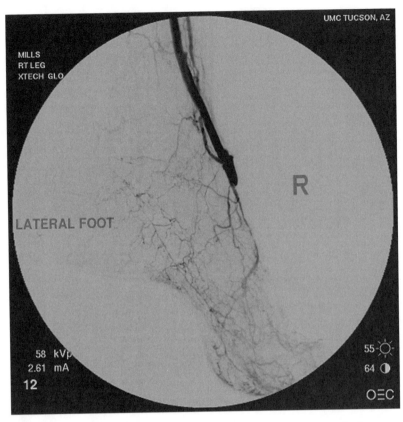

Figure 11.2 Completion arteriogram of the same patient after reversed vein bypass to the dorsalis pedis artery (dpa). Despite occlusive disease in the distal dpa, the toe amputation healed (great toe pressure improved to 65 mmHg after the bypass), and the graft has remained patent for >1 year. The patient wears protective footwear and has had no recurrent foot lesions.

result of persistent, unfounded myths and commonly held misconceptions: *1*) gangrene results from microvascular disease, *2*) foot incisions don't heal in patients with diabetes, and *3*) bypasses don't work as well in patients with diabetes.

Abundant clinical data over the last decades have proved that none of these myths is true. Clinically important lower-extremity ischemia in patients with diabetes mellitus is caused by arteriosclerosis, and the disease pattern can usually be corrected by revascularization. Diabetic patients with foot lesions and diminished or absent foot pulses, or those who fail to heal despite apparently adequate circulation, should promptly be referred to an experienced vascular surgeon. Noninvasive testing and liberal use of arteriography allows significant vascular lesions to be identified and corrected. Endovascular approaches are occasionally appropriate, but a surgical option for revascularization is available in nearly every case. Revascularization results in 75–80% limb salvage at five years (15,19). Early referral and aggressive revascularization are likely to substantially reduce the number of unnecessary major limb amputations (20).

References

1. Strandness DE: Diabetes mellitus and vascular surgery. In *Basic Data Underlying Clinical Decision Making in Vascular Surgery.* Porter JM, Taylor LM. St. Louis, MO, Quality Medical Publishing, 1994, p. 30–33

2. American Diabetes Association: Peripheral arterial disease in people with diabetes (Position Statement). *Diabetes Care* 26:3333–3341, 2003

3. Pomposelli FB, Domenig C: Diabetic foot problems. In *Comprehensive Vascular and Endovascular Surgery.* Hallett JW, Mills JL, Earnshaw JJ, Reekers JA, Eds. New York, Elsevier, 2004, p. 177–188

4. Strandness DE, Priest RE, Gibbons GE: Combined clinical and pathologic study of diabetic and nondiabetic peripheral arterial disease. *Diabetes* 13:366–372, 1964

5. Beach KW, Brunzell JD, Strandness DE Jr: Prevalence of severe arteriosclerosis obliterans in patients with diabetes mellitus: relation to smoking and form of therapy. *Arteriosclerosis* 2:275–280, 1982

6. Beach KW, Brunzell JD, Conquest LL, Strandness DE: The correlation of arteriosclerosis obliterans with lipoproteins in insulin-dependent and non-insulin-dependent diabetes. *Diabetes* 28:836–840, 1979

7. Beach KW, Strandness DE Jr: Arteriosclerosis obliterans and associated risk factors in insulin-dependent and non-insulin-dependent diabetes. *Diabetes* 29:882–888, 1980

8. Beach KW, Bedford GR, Bergelin RO, Martin DC, Vandenberghe N, Zaccardi M, Strandness DE Jr: Progression of lower-extremity arterial occlusive disease in type II diabetes mellitus. *Diabetes Care* 11:464–472, 1988

9. LoGerfo FW, Coffman JD: Vascular and microvascular disease of the foot in diabetes. *N Engl J Med* 311:1615–1618, 1984

10. Goldenberg S, Alex M, Joshi RA, Blumenthal, HT: Nonatheromatous peripheral vascular disease of the lower extremity in diabetes mellitus. *Diabetes* 8:261–273, 1959

11. Akbari CM, Pomposelli FB Jr, Gibbons GW, Campbell DR, Pulling MC, Mydlarz D, LoGerfo FW: Lower extremity revascularization in diabetes: late observations. *Arch Surg* 135:452–456, 2000

12. Johnson BL, Glickman MH, Bandyk DF, Esses GE: Failure of foot salvage in patients with end-stage renal disease after surgical revascularization. *J Vasc Surg* 22:280–285, discussion 285–286, 1995

13. Weitz JI, Byrne J, Clagett GP, Farkouh ME, Porter JM, Sackett DL, Strandness DE Jr, Taylor LM: Diagnosis and treatment of chronic arterial insufficiency of the lower extremities: a critical review [see erratum in *Circulation* 102:1074, 2000]. *Circulation* 94:3026–3049, 1996

14. Gentile AT, Berman SS, Reinke KR, Demas CP, Ihnat DH, Hughes JD, Mills JL: A regional pedal ischemia scoring system for decision analysis in patients with heel ulceration. *Am J Surg* 176:109–114, 1998

15. Taylor LM Jr, Porter JM: Results of lower extremity bypass in the diabetic patient. *Sem Vasc Surg* 5:226–233, 1992

16. Mills JL, Gahtan V, Fujitani R, Taylor SM, Bandyk DF: The utility and durability of vein bypass grafts originating from the popliteal artery for limb salvage. *Am J Surg* 168:646–651, 1994

17. Pomposelli FB Jr, Jepsen SJ, Gibbons GW, Campbell DR, Freeman DV, Miller A, LoGerfo FW: Efficacy of the dorsal pedal bypass for limb salvage in diabetic patients: short term observations. *J Vasc Surg* 11:745–751, 1990

18. Tannenbaum GA, Pomposelli FB Jr, Marcaccio EJ, Gibbons GW, Campbell DR, Freeman DV, Miller A, LoGerfo FW: Safety of vein bypass grafting to the dorsal pedal artery in diabetic patients with foot infections. *J Vasc Surg* 15:982–990, 1992

19. Taylor LM Jr, Porter JM: The clinical course of diabetics who require emergent foot surgery because of infection or ischemia. *J Vasc Surg* 6:454–459, 1987

20. Mills JL, Beckett WC, Taylor SM: The diabetic foot: consequences of delayed treatment and referral. *South Med J* 84:970–974, 1991

Index

symptoms, 79–82
x-rays for, 80
Charcot neuroarthropathy (CN).
    See Charcot foot
Charcot's joint disease. *See* Charcot
    foot
Chopart amputations, 71
Chronic wounds, 2–9
  acute wound pathophysiology,
    2–4
  adjunctive therapies. *See*
    Adjunctive wound therapies
  cardinal defects of, 4–5
  debridement of. *See*
    Debridement
  foot ulcers. *See* Foot ulcers
  moderate infections, 95
  pathophysiology of, 5
  wound hypoxia, 6
Claw toes, 13, 16, 48
Coagulation, 2
Coagulum, debriding, 66–67
Compliance issues
  footwear, 42–43
  off-loading of foot wounds,
    57–58
Contamination, wound, 91
Critical limb ischemia, 46–47
Crutches, 53
Custom footwear, 39–40
Custom insoles, 41

D

Debridement, 61–71
  of acute wounds, 61
  aggressive, 62
  to avoid amputation, 71

of bone, 69–70
of chronic wounds, 61
of fascia, 68–69
hydrosurgical debrider, 63
infected wound assessment and,
    93
with maggots, 70
of muscle, 69
nonsurgical modes of, 70
postdebridement care, 70–71
repeated, of nonhealing ischemic
    foot, 101
of skin, 68
of subcutaneous tissue, 68
surgical, 63–70
of tendons, 69
timing of, 62
tools for, 63
topical enzymatic debriding
    agents, 70
wet-to-dry dressings, 70
wound healing and, 61–62
Depth inlay shoes, 39, 53–54
Dermagraft, 75
Dermatologic examination, 19, 21
DH Pressure Relief Walker, 56
Diabetic foot team, 34
Diabetic microangiopathy, myth
    of, 100
Diabetic wounds, healing of, 5–9.
    See also Foot ulcers; Infection,
    diabetic foot
Digital waveform/pressure mea-
    surements, 101
Discoloration, 46
Distal symmetric peripheral
    neuropathy. *See* Peripheral
    neuropathy

reducing, 9
Inflammatory pathways, 8–9
Insoles, 40, 41
Instant total contact cast, 57, 58
International Working Group on the Diabetic Foot (IWGDF), 24, 32–34
Ischemic ulcers, 29
  assessing, 46–47
  location of, 47
  repeated debridement of, 101

J

Joint mobility, limited, 24
  as Charcot foot risk factor, 82
  foot deformities and, 30
  inflammatory excess and, 9
  neuropathy and, 7

L

Lisfranc amputations, 71
Low-adherent dressings, 73
Lower-extremity bypass, 102

M

MABAL shoe, 54
Macrovascular disease, 6, 7
Maggots, as debriding agent, 70
Magnetic resonance imaging (MRI)
  Charcot foot assessment, 84
  infected wound assessment, 93
  osteomyelitis diagnosis, 48, 95
Mechanical trauma, 16, 31

Medicaid, HBO reimbursement, 76
Medicare
  footwear benefit, 42, 43
  HBO reimbursements, 76
Meggitt-Wagner classification system, 48–49
Metatarsal heads, prominent, 13, 16, 48
  healing sandals and, 53–54
Microvascular disease, 6, 8
Mild infections, 92, 94, 96
Moderate infections, 92, 94–95, 96
Muscle, debridement of, 69

N

Neuroischemic ulcers, 46, 47
Neuropathic osteoarthropathy. *See* Charcot foot
Neuropathic ulcers, 29, 47
Neuropathy
  amputation and, 2
  autonomic. *See* Autonomic neuropathy
  calluses and, 7
  foot deformities and, 6–7
  as foot ulcer risk factor, 12–13, 16
  limited joint mobility and, 6–7
  peripheral. *See* Peripheral neuropathy
  polyneuropathy, 48
  screening for, 19, 21–23, 29, 48
  somatic, 13, 15
NFκB, 8–9
Noncontact normothermic wound therapy (NNWT), 77

T

Technetium bone scans, 84
Tendons, debridement of, 69
Therapeutic footwear. *See*
 Footwear
Thermal trauma, 16
Tinea pedis, 21
Toe-brachial index, 46
Toenails
 examining, 21
 paronychia, 92
Toe pressure measurements, 46
 PAD screening, 30, 101
Topical enzymatic debriding
 agents, 70
Topical radiant heat (TRH) ther-
 apy, 77
Total contact casts, 55–56
Transcutaneous oxygen pressure
 (tcPO$_2$), 30, 46
Trauma
 amputation and, 2
 as Charcot foot risk factor, 82,
 83
 mechanical, 16, 31
 puncture injuries, 31
 thermal, 16
Tuning forks, 22, 48

U

University of Texas (UT) classification system, 48–49

V

Vacuum-assisted closure (VAC),
 69, 75–76
Vascular disease, 7–8
Vascular examination, 23, 30, 46
Vein grafts, 102
Vibration perception threshold
 (VPT), 22–23, 29

W

Walkers, 53
Warm foot, 16, 46, 83
Warm-Up (TRH therapy), 77
WBC imaging, 84
Wedges, 39
Wet gangrene, 62
Wet-to-dry dressings, 70
Wheelchairs, 53
Wound hypoxia, 6, 7–8
Wounds
 acute. *See* Acute wounds
 chronic. *See* Chronic wounds;
 Foot ulcers
 healing of. *See* Adjunctive
 wound therapies; Healing
 infected. *See* Infection, diabetic
 foot

X

X-rays
 Charcot foot, 80, 81, 83
 infected wound, 93
 osteomyelitis, 47–48

About the American Diabetes Association

The American Diabetes Association is the nation's leading voluntary health organization supporting diabetes research, information, and advocacy. Its mission is to prevent and cure diabetes and to improve the lives of all people affected by diabetes. The American Diabetes Association is the leading publisher of comprehensive diabetes information. Its huge library of practical and authoritative books for people with diabetes covers every aspect of self-care—cooking and nutrition, fitness, weight control, medications, complications, emotional issues, and general self-care.

To order American Diabetes Association books: Call 1-800-232-6733. Or log on to http://store.diabetes.org

To join the American Diabetes Association: Call 1-800-806-7801. www.diabetes.org/membership

For more information about diabetes or ADA programs and services: Call 1-800-342-2383. E-mail: AskADA@diabetes.org or log on to www.diabetes.org

To locate an ADA/NCQA Recognized Provider of quality diabetes care in your area: www.ncqa.org/dprp

To find an ADA Recognized Education Program in your area: Call 1-888-232-0822. www.diabetes.org/recognition/education.asp

To join the fight to increase funding for diabetes research, end discrimination, and improve insurance coverage: Call 1-800-342-2383. www.diabetes.org/advocacy

To find out how you can get involved with the programs in your community: Call 1-800-342-2383. See below for program Web addresses.

- *American Diabetes Month:* educational activities aimed at those diagnosed with diabetes—month of November. www.diabetes.org/ADM
- *American Diabetes Alert:* annual public awareness campaign to find the undiagnosed—held the fourth Tuesday in March. www.diabetes.org/alert
- *The Diabetes Assistance & Resources Program (DAR):* diabetes awareness program targeted to the Latino community. www.diabetes.org/DAR
- *African American Program:* diabetes awareness program targeted to the African American community. www.diabetes.org/africanamerican
- *Awakening the Spirit: Pathways to Diabetes Prevention & Control:* diabetes awareness program targeted to the Native American community. www.diabetes.org/awakening

To find out about an important research project regarding type 2 diabetes: www.diabetes.org/ada/research.asp

To obtain information on making a planned gift or charitable bequest: Call 1-888-700-7029. www.diabetes.org/ada/plan.asp

To make a donation or memorial contribution: Call 1-800-342-2383. www.diabetes.org/ada/cont.asp